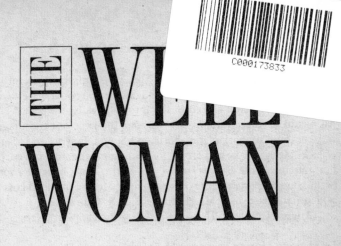

THE WELL WOMAN

Dr MARGERY MORGAN

BBC Books

AUTHOR'S ACKNOWLEDGEMENTS

Barry Lynch of BBC Wales started this all – I'm very grateful for his vision and advice. Thanks, too, to Jennifer Jones, who worked with such interest and enthusiasm to help realise the book.

All would have been impossible without the generous encouragement and constant support of my husband, Simon Emery, and thanks to Jack, Holly, Blaise and Henry for sparing me the time and energy.

I'm grateful to the *British Journal of Obstetrics and Gynaecology* for their permission to reproduce the 'Assessment of Menstrual Blood Loss Using a Pictorial Chart' by J.M. Higham, P.M.S. O'Brien and R.W. Shaw (August 1990, vol.97, pages 734–9) which appears on page 48.

Dr Margery Morgan trained at Sheffield University Medical School and is currently Senior Registrar in Obstetrics and Gynaecology at Singleton Hospital, Swansea. She has produced health programmes for Saudi Arabian radio and was the presenter for the BBC Radio Derby *Well-Woman* series. She is married to a consultant gynaecologist, they have four children and live in Wales.

Published by BBC Books,
a division of BBC Enterprises Limited,
Woodlands, 80 Wood Lane, London W12 0TT
First published 1992
Reprinted 1992
© Dr Margery Morgan 1992
ISBN 0 563 36307 X
Designed by Grahame Dudley Associates
Illustrations by Kate Simunek
Set in Garamond 3 Roman by Goodfellow & Egan, Cambridge
Printed and bound in Great Britain by Clays Ltd, St Ives plc
Cover printed by Clays Ltd, St Ives plc

This book accompanies the series *Health UK The Well-Woman*, made by Prospect Pictures for BBC Wales and BBC1. The series was first broadcast on BBC1 in the spring of 1992.

CONTENTS

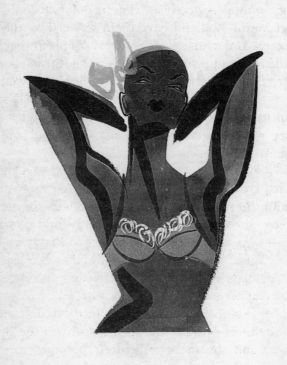

FOREWORD

It is very tempting to think of our bodies as machines, capable of running perfectly in tune if only we could find the correct petrol-food and have them serviced by the best garage-doctor. Unfortunately it is not as simple as that, and the very idea of an optimum 'wellness' is an illusion – every state of health is subjective and relative, and one woman's meat can literally be another woman's poison. Diseases are not entities separate from the bodies that suffer from them: they are reactions between the individual and her environment.

The modern woman, however, is no longer prepared to put up with conditions of health that fall too short of her idea of how she should feel, and neither will she let the doctors keep all their information hidden behind screens of medical mystique and jargon. She wants to know, to have the facts explained to her and to be allowed to take part, as far as any layman can, in any interpretations and decisions involved in diagnosis and treatment.

The more complex and varied medical knowledge becomes, the more options are open in turn to the doctor and patient, and the more difficult it becomes to make judgements on the appropriate course of action. A good, common sense appreciation of the workings of the body can help the patient faced with a change in her health – whether caused by a welcome pregnancy or the onslaught of disease – to approach it with intelligence and without fear, and the emergence of new contagious and incurable viral diseases now means that an understanding of basic preventive medicine is no longer just desirable but essential.

Gone are the days when mysterious 'women's problems' were subjects unsuitable for discussion even in the privacy of our own homes, only to be mentioned in excited wide-eyed whispers in the school lavatories. We are in an age of openness and frankness, when HRT can be discussed at the dinner table and period pains on the bus. This welcome state of openness, along with the urge to 'know our own bodies', has also proved a fertile ground for the birth of self-help remedies and optimistic offers of paths to super-health. While some alternative therapies may be helpful, such as homeopathy and acupuncture, others have yet to be proved of benefit.

In *The Well-Woman*, Dr Morgan presents us with a sensible, clear analysis of what we need to know about ourselves to try to keep healthy without fanaticism or worry. We have the opportunity now more than ever before to make considered decisions about our bodies and how we treat them. Whether this book is read straight through or dipped into as a work of reference, it will serve to increase the realistic knowledge upon which such decisions must be based.

JANE ASHER

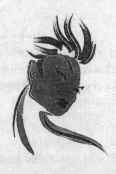

—1—
THE WELL-WOMAN

Woman today have more opportunity to take responsibility for their health, and to take control of their bodies. They are also better informed about how their bodies work in general. Hopefully, gone are the days when a young girl started her periods in complete ignorance, when jokes in the playground were often the only guide to sex and birth control, and when childbirth was a terrifying voyage into the unknown. Knowing what to expect, say with our periods or a first pregnancy, is both reassuring and alerts us to when things aren't right and advice is needed. Examining our breasts at home is also a good idea for picking up problems early on, when the chances of a cure are far higher.

We need to be as well informed as possible about the health checks available for women. Some family doctors and family planning clinics are now offering a well-woman service, which includes regular cervical smears and other tests. If anything should be wrong, it's also good to know what treatment is involved; especially if it could be something serious, not knowing can create unnecessary fear and tension.

Taking control of our lives, maintaining a healthy lifestyle with a good diet and frequent exercise, will give us the best chance of staying fit, looking good and feeling happy.

Who'd be a woman?
This may come as a surprise to some women, but we are physically the stronger sex. For a start, we have to be in order to cope with the whole business of bearing children. This begins at birth: if there are two ill babies, one of each sex, in a special care unit, the girl has a better chance of survival. Our nicely balanced XX chromosomes (the chromosomes that determined our sex at conception) seem to give us a stabilising advantage. This means that any condition carried on one of the X chromosomes, like the gene for colour blindness or haemophilia, is balanced out by the normal X chromosome. The woman then becomes a carrier of the condition. (If both chromosomes were affected the fetus wouldn't survive. If a male baby inherits the faulty X chromosome then he gets the condition.)

Many of us are privileged to experience the joy of having a baby, including the peculiar sensation of someone hiccoughing inside us or giving the most stomach-aching kicks. Then there are the overwhelming feelings of love for the baby, which make the hard bits of pregnancy, giving birth and looking after someone so dependent on us worthwhile. And not to mention feeding a baby from the breast. All quite amazing!

Because of our hormones, we have much less chance of having a heart attack than men until we reach the menopause, when things tend to even out. On average, we also live five years longer than men. At the same time, because of our complex and delicate reproductive system, we spend more time at the doctor's and in hospitals than men. So it is important to look after ourselves, and to follow a well-woman life plan.

GOOD HEALTH GUIDELINES

A healthy lifestyle gives us the best chance of staying fit and well. This means paying attention to our diet, keeping in touch with the news on what's good for us, and eating lots of low fat, high fibre foods, with plenty of fresh fruit and vegetables. It also means taking some form of regular exercise.

Avoiding poisons, such as tobacco and alcohol in excess, is essential for optimum health. Although most of us know it is madness to smoke, it is an addiction that is very difficult to stop. Giving up successfully often means getting lots of help and support. Like losing weight, the people who are most successful at giving up smoking are those who have done it as part of a group. Everyone gives each other the sympathy and encouragement to go on. (For more details, see page 15.)

Alcohol isn't so much of a problem if taken in moderation, but it is addictive for some people, and in excess and over a long period of time it can cause serious damage to the mind and body. Remember that women should always drink less than men – our bodies are not so well equipped to take alcohol. (For more details, see page 14.)

DIET AND DIETING

Many woman have a love-hate relationship with their bodies. At any one time, one woman in seven is on a diet. We want to look our best, and take time and care over our appearance, only to get depressed over what we see as our physical faults. Part of the problem is that we are constantly exposed to images of the perfect woman (young, slender and with striking looks), particularly in advertisements in magazines, on television and in the cinema. There are two basic messages: the first is buy this product and, like her, you will be desirable, young, slim, exciting, etc.; the second is that this woman represents all women; that is, young, desirable, slim, exciting, etc. So whether we buy that particular product or not, when we don't match up we feel guilty and miserable. A few facts might help to put things into perspective.

An important fact is that these models do not have much to do with reality. They are often teenagers who have exceptional looks, and who have been carefully made-up and groomed for the occasion. It is their job to look glamorous and poised for the camera, and there is a whole team of people – make-up artists, lighting cameramen, stylists – to make sure that they do. The finished product represents, at most, a few moments in time – no one in real life, however well groomed, can carry on without getting the odd crumple in her clothes, or a shiny nose, or a hair out of place. And that's before the airbrush artist steps in to cover up any blemishes on the photograph itself!

The other problem is that we may criticise our own bodies as a way of diverting feelings of anger and frustration about other areas of our lives. No one has to tell us how destructive this can be. In such cases, we need to look at the real problems, not take it out on our bodies. It may also help to realise that women come in all shapes and sizes – thin, fat, medium, big-bottomed, small-breasted, busty – that this is normal, and that the happiest ones are those who have accepted and esteem themselves for what they are.

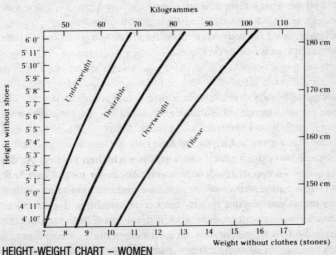

HEIGHT-WEIGHT CHART – WOMEN

What is overweight?
To work out whether your weight is average for your height, overweight or seriously fat (obese), divide your weight in kilograms (W) by your height in metres (H) times itself (1 in = 0.0254 m, 1 lb = 0.45 kg). This is the body mass index. For example, if you weigh 60 kilograms and you measure 1.7 metres, your body mass index = 60/1.7 x 1.7 = 20.76. Between 20 and 24.9 is desirable; 25 to 29.9 is overweight, and over 30 is seriously overweight, or obese. (If you've lost your calculator, use the height/weight chart on page 9.)

Many women complain that even staying reasonably slim is a constant battle. The usual story is a gradual increase in weight from the twenties to middle age. (This is true for men as well as women.) This is caused by any number of life events: having children and losing sight of our image during and after pregnancy, spending time in the kitchen producing solid meals for the starving hordes, using food as a comfort device, taking less exercise and/or having a sedentary job. The menopause also seems to make some women put on weight. It may also be partly due to inherited body type. Endomorphs are more prone naturally to put on weight and have difficulty losing it: they tend to be short, with round bodies and wide hips. Their hands and feet are often small and delicate. Ectomorphs, on the other hand, are naturally slim, with long limbs, but less stamina. They rarely have problems keeping their weight down. The last type, the mesomorphs, have naturally athletic builds, with strong shoulders and narrow hips. They seem to have lots of energy, and not much of a weight problem.

A monthly check on your weight should tell you if you need to take care and restrict intake of certain foods.

LOSING WEIGHT
There are positive health reasons for losing excess weight – it will help to reduce your chances of suffering from heart disease, diabetes, gall-stones, high blood pressure, and even arthritis. But it is now well known that dieting can make you fat! It's the way we lose weight that is important. A low-calorie diet, where you are starving your body (the World Health Organisation defines starvation as an intake of 1,000 calories or less a day) will result in rapid weight loss. However, unless you then revise your eating habits, the excess weight will go straight back on once you stop the diet. Faddy diets often lead to bingeing because the body is desperate for vital nutrients (a high protein diet can lead to a craving for carbohydrates – particularly before a period – for

example). Strict diets can also leave you feeling bored, apathetic and generally feeling low. Even worse, constant dieting can slow your natural metabolism down (the rate at which you use up calories) – in effect, your body eventually learns to function on less calories. The result is that you have to eat even less to maintain your ideal weight, and you can get caught up in a spiral of self deprivation and misery.

The solution is change the way you eat – preferably forever – and at the same time to take up some regular form of exercise that you enjoy (page 12). (Regular exercise not only helps you to stay fit. It replaces fat with muscle tissue, and muscle tissue burns more calories than fat.) The diet guidelines set out in the next section (see below) give you all the basic information you need for both a weight reduction regime and a healthy eating plan for life. Based on the World Health Organisation's recommendations, it emphasises the importance of carbohydrate foods (not often considered the dieter's friend), as well as plenty of fresh fruit and vegetables. Carbohydrates release their sugar more slowly, ensuring a steady level of sugar in the blood, which means you won't feel tired or hungry between meals. You will lose weight slowly on this diet (between 450 g/1 lb and 1 kg/2 lb a week), but it should stay off. If you are beginning to feel deprived, it's better to allow yourself the occasional sweet or cake (a form of treat allowance) than to risk losing your self-control later on and giving up completely. If you do have a weak moment, don't turn this into a failure – just accept that it's done and continue with the diet. It's best not to weigh yourself every day (body water fluctuates day by day), especially if your are overconcerned about losing weight. You might prefer to monitor your weight loss with a tape measure instead.

If you are seriously overweight (see chart on page 9), see your GP.

THE BALANCED DIET

The low fat, high fibre diet is the one recommended in the World Health Organisation's recent international report, 'Diet, Nutrition and the Prevention of Chronic Disease'. This will help to reduce heart disease, prevent cancer, improve bowel disorders, and a host of other less serious, everyday ailments.

The WHO guidelines are as follows:

Fats We must reduce all fats – saturated, monounsaturated and polyunsaturated – in our diet, but especially saturated fats. This means eating vegetable margarines instead of butter, reducing our intake of red meat (eat poultry and fish instead), and cutting down on milk, cream and cheese. Most of us would benefit from reducing our fat intake by at least a third to a half (that is, no more than 30 per cent of our energy – calories – should come from fats and oils of all types).

When eating meat, choose lean cuts, avoid pies and sausages (even low fat ones) because of their very high fat content, and always grill or dry roast meat. Better still, go for chicken, turkey or fish instead. Oily fish like mackerel or sardines, which are high in healthy polyunsaturates, may have a protective effect on the heart and arteries.

Hard cheeses, like Cheddar, are high in fat; soft cheeses are better for you, and less fattening, especially cottage cheese. Adults should change from full-fat milk to skimmed or semi-skimmed versions, but this is not recommended for children under five.

Fibre Fresh fruit, vegetables and unrefined starchy foods – wholemeal bread, brown rice, lentils and wholemeal pasta – are high in fibre. The WHO recommends we should eat about five portions of fruit and vegetables every day, and starchy foods should represent 50–70 per cent of our calories. Most of us should double our intake of starchy foods.

Drinks Alcohol is fairly high in calories but low in nutrients, so cut down if you're watching your weight and for health generally (page 14). Drink orange juice, or any fruit juice which is enriched with Vitamin C – this increases the iron available to the body, which is very necessary for all menstruating women, especially vegetarians. Don't overdose on tea and coffee: both are powerful stimulants and can have some unpleasant side-effects such as palpitations, anxiety and insomnia. Fizzy drinks are loaded with calories and not much else. Go for herb teas, mineral water or fruit juices diluted with water instead.

Problem foods We must cut down on empty foods, such as sweets, cakes, biscuits, sugary soft drinks, ice cream and sugar itself. Sugar is high in calories, but offers almost no nutrients. It makes weight control difficult if there is already a problem, and is a major contributor to tooth decay. The WHO recommends that sugar, in any form, should represent no more than 10 per cent of our calorie intake. For most people, this means cutting our consumption by half.

EXERCISE FOR FUN

Exercise has a lot going for it. A variety of exercise keeps us looking trim, helps control weight, strengthens the heart and lungs, and builds up bones. Unfortunately, it is not always easy to find time to exercise if we have full-time jobs, or growing families to look after. Our more sedentary lifestyle doesn't help either – the car has made us all so lazy, and walking is no longer a part of the normal day.

Aerobic exercise is the best way of keeping fit and trim; it tones the circulation, the heart and the lungs. This is the kind of exercise that gets you out of breath, where you are using the muscles of your arms and legs. To be good for you the exercise needs to be vigorous enough that you'd find keeping up a conversation turns into a breathy chat. Aerobic exercise includes walking, jogging, squash and swimming.

Anaerobic exercise is where you make your muscles contract but don't necessarily get out of breath. This includes weight lifting, isometric exercises and yoga, which are all good for building either strength or suppleness.

British research has looked at the effect of twenty minutes' exercise four to five times a week. This managed to reduce blood pressure and pulse rates in the people studied, as well as lowering blood cholesterol. Once the exercise was stopped the effects wore off. So the benefits of exercise come from regular frequent activity, little and often, for life.

Measuring fitness

You can overdo exercising, especially if you are over thirty-five, over-weight and never normally do any physical activity. Your heart will respond to the increased demands of your muscles to supply them with more oxygen. To do this, it has to beat faster and so your pulse rate goes up. If it goes up too much you will be putting additional strain on the heart and you will need to slow down.

To make sure you are exercising at the right level for you, check your pulse rate immediately after ten minutes of strenuous exercise (feel with two fingers on the thumb side of the wrist). Count your pulse for ten seconds and multiply it by six to get your rate. If it's above your allowed maximum you are doing too much too soon, if it's below the minimum you can work harder.

Recommended pulse rate per minute after exercise		
Age	Minimum	Maximum
20–29	140	170
30–39	130	160
40–49	125	140
50–59	115	130
60–69	105	120

You will soon work out how much you can safely do, and the more you exercise the stronger your heart will be.

PUTTING IT INTO PRACTICE

Make exercise part of your new lifestyle. If it's practical, take the stairs, instead of the lift, walk to the shops, volunteer to do the errands, take the dog for a walk. Enjoy being on the move. In addition, try to take some regular physical activity. Some women prefer to exercise alone, others prefer the support of a group. Try swimming or jogging if you're a solitary exerciser. For some women having a fixed arrangement – a keep-fit or aerobics class or tennis with a friend – makes it more difficult to cancel and makes exercising much more enjoyable. Disco dancing, cycling or badminton are all excellent forms of exercise.

Fitting this in can be difficult. Look at your schedule: have you time to exercise in the mornings before work, do you have any time without the kids in the week? If you're stuck at home, with no transport or babysitter, then try creating an exercise plan for yourself and stick to it. One of the fitness videos may help to get you going. Or try skipping, building up to ten minutes a day (that's quite a long time).

WOMEN AND ALCOHOL

Women are more susceptible to alcohol than men. Proportionally, we contain less water in our bodies; this means we become intoxicated more quickly and suffer the long-term effects of alcohol abuse sooner than any man. Alcohol is a poison to the liver and to a growing fetus. The recommended alcohol limit for women is 14 units per week. A unit equals a glass of wine; or 300 ml/½ pint of beer, lager or cider; or a single measure of spirits. (Men are allowed 3 units a day because of their bigger liver and different metabolism.)

When we drink, alcohol is absorbed into the bloodstream, sometimes making us feel relaxed and happy, sometimes gloomy and depressed – all the time it is blunting the brain's functions and performance. We're then not so good at coordination and certainly can't drive competently (most women who drink more than 3–4 units in one hour will be over the legal limit – that is, a blood alcohol level of over 80mg/100ml). The liver has to cope with getting rid of most of the alcohol – converting it to acetaldehyde – at the expense of its normal functions. In other words, alcohol can interfere with the proper metabolism of fat, protein and glucose. This is made even worse if meals are skipped and drinks taken instead.

Women seem to get more cirrhosis of the liver than men – this is the change in the liver from normal functioning cells to scar-like fibrous tissue – although some people are more susceptible than others. Steady drinkers are apparently more at risk than binge drinkers. Alcohol has been mentioned in the debate over breast cancer – one study said it increased your chances of contracting the disease, another said it didn't. Liver cancer, however, is more common if the liver has already been damaged by alcohol.

In pregnancy

When you are pregnant, alcohol passes from your bloodstream through the placenta to the baby's circulation. Babies whose mothers drink excessively in pregnancy can develop *fetal alcohol syndrome*: they are born with a broad flat face and a flattened nose, and are sometimes also mentally retarded. Most of these babies have been born in America and France to mothers with a high alcohol intake (200 ml/7 fl oz of spirits a day). Cannabis and opium seem to produce similar effects. The syndrome is not wholly due to alcohol as it appears more often in babies of lower income mothers than in those of middle-class mothers – the effects of a poor diet and cigarette smoking may contribute as well.

Even small amounts of alcohol may cause problems with fetal growth, so the current advice is to avoid alcohol altogether or limit your intake to less than four drinks a week in pregnancy. Pregnant women should never get drunk as it's binge drinking that's thought to be more harmful to the baby.

If you are thinking about getting pregnant cut down your alcohol intake or give up now. In fetal growth the first days and weeks are the most important in terms of organ development, and this could be at a time when you don't even know you are pregnant. Heavy drinking can also double your risk of miscarriage.

Alcohol Concern, 305 Grays Inn Road, London WC1X 8QF. Tel: 071–833 3471.
Alcoholics Anonymous, 11 Redcliffe Gardens, London SW10 9BG. Tel: 071-352 3001. For information and details of groups in your area contact Al Anon Family Groups, 61 Dover Street, London SE1 4YF. Tel: 071–403 0888.

WOMEN AND SMOKING

Despite all the publicity about the harmful effects of smoking more women than ever are taking up the habit. The number of teenage girls who are smoking is also increasing. Younger women may take up smoking to signal maturity and independence; unfortunately, nicotine is a highly addictive, and poisonous, drug which is very difficult to control. Stress may also play a part in why women smoke. The problem has reached such a scale that lung cancer has nearly overtaken breast cancer as the most common cancer in women.

Smoking trebles our chances of getting heart disease even though our hormones protect us during the years we are menstruating. Women smokers have an earlier menopause, so they lose their valuable oestrogen hormones sooner.

Lung cancer is on the increase in women, and 90 per cent of cases are caused by smoking. Smoking breaks down the lining of the lung passages which is why smokers are prone to chest infections such as chronic bronchitis and emphysema. Smoking also has an effect on the cervix, bringing an increased chance of cervical cancer. It makes taking the oral contraceptive pill more dangerous, too.

If you give up smoking today your risks of having a heart attack come down almost straight away. The lung cancer risk drops more slowly (it takes between ten and fifteen years to reach the risk levels of a non-smoker), but other chest problems usually improve quickly.

'Passive smoking', inhaling other people's cigarette smoke, is also a serious problem, and for this reason more and more public places are becoming smoke-free zones. Regular exposure to passive smoking in adults increases their chances of lung cancer, and children have a greater chance of chest infections and asthma.

SMOKING AND THE LUNGS

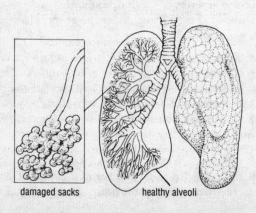

damaged sacks   healthy alveoli

In pregnancy

It is well known that babies of women who smoke are smaller and that the number of failed pregnancies overall is much greater in smokers. Carbon monoxide, which is increased in smokers' blood, gets through to the baby and affects the haemoglobin's oxygen-carrying ability. Nicotine causes the blood vessels of the placenta to get narrower (as it does in adult blood vessels) and this reduces the amount of blood feeding through to the placenta for the baby. This effect may be made worse by drinking lots of coffee – smokers usually drink coffee and, as the caffeine acts in a similar way to nicotine, it is a damaging combination. It takes longer for caffeine to be metabolised in pregnancy, which may add to the problem. Certainly, smokers who give up cigarettes need to cut down their coffee drinking at the same time because of this effect on the metabolism.

The advice to a prospective mother must be to give up smoking now and forever.

Ash, Action on Smoking and Health, 109 Gloucester Place, London W1H 3DA. Tel: 071-935 3519.
QUIT: Smoker's quit line. Tel: 071-487 3000.

WOMEN AND MENTAL HEALTH

Depression is particularly common in women, and many women complain about the amount of stress and anxiety they experience in their lives. Men also suffer from these problems, but for most women who have been brought up to be the nurturing, sensitive sex, it can be especially hard to find the right balance in an industrialised society where employment and financial independence are highly valued. Girls are brought up to be wives and mothers, carers of children, the aged and the handicapped, and are expected to put others' needs before their own, often in isolation and with little recognition from society (and certainly very little financial support or other benefits). This can lead to irritability, frustration and despair. Because they are not encouraged to express their anger and frustration, it is common for women to internalise these; this can lead to mental distress. Women from minority racial groups may also suffer from stereotyping, harassment and problems in getting the right help and support because of language difficulties and cultural differences. Qualities that are encouraged in young boys, such as assertiveness, aggression and independence, are not seen as appropriate in young girls. When women are then asked to join the workforce, often because of economic forces, they cannot always bring qualities that are respected in a male-dominated world. It's no wonder then that there is a conflict between society's changing expectations of what women should be and do and how women see themselves. These dilemmas can cause unhappiness, and sometimes they can result in mental illness.

If women stay at home, there may be a part of them that always stays dependent. If their partners abandon them or die, or cannot provide for them any longer, there is financial and emotional distress; even the fear that this might happen can cause stress. Being a mother is stressful enough in itself, even when there is adequate support. Single women have to provide for themselves; if they put their careers before everything else, there may come a point where they will regret not finding a partner and having children (and they may ask themselves, 'Should I have done that anyway?'). Working mothers and single parents have to juggle family needs with those of their jobs. And as women become old and can no longer work or have children, they may feel unwanted, unwillingly dependent and unattractive; practically, they may face poverty, discrimination and isolation.

STRESS

A certain amount of stress in our lives is normal, even beneficial. It can be stimulating, even invigorating. But beyond a certain point stress can affect our physical and mental wellbeing. If we are faced with more stress than we can cope with the sympathetic nervous system is activated, preparing for action by producing adrenaline. The pulse rate goes up, breathing gets faster, blood pressure goes up and blood is diverted to the muscles. This is known as the 'fight or flight' mechanism. The problems we have to deal with today seldom require physical activity, which leaves you feeling tense, with a pounding heart and indigestion.

Short-term stress tends to occur in one-off situations – going to the dentist, having a minor accident, the house being burgled. These are situations that can be dealt with there and then.

Long-term stress is more difficult to cope with, such as partnership problems, a serious illness, even getting married or pregnancy. This may call up continuous stress responses.

Stress can make you more susceptible to infection, and can eventually lead to more serious conditions such as duodenal ulcers, arthritis, asthma and colitis. Women can also suffer from menstrual problems, sexual difficulties, failure to ovulate, amenorrhoea and infertility.

The symptoms of stress can include compulsive eating, menstrual disorders, headaches, stomach pains, either insomnia or a desire to sleep all the time, and palpitations.

How can stress be dealt with?

Although it may not always be easy, distancing yourself from the stressful situation will help. It is very difficult to think clearly in the 'fight or flight' state. Is there anyone you can go to for advice or help? To get things into perspective you might try sitting down and first defining the problem, then writing out all the choices you have and opting for a realistic solution. If possible, make an action plan to follow through. Try not to worry or dwell on situations in the past or the future; worry like this can be habit forming, and will do nothing for your stress levels. There are also practical, self-help measures you can take to help minimise the effects of stress.

EXERCISE This is one of the best ways of relieving stress (page 12).

RELAXATION TECHNIQUES Deep breathing and relaxation will help you to switch off. Lie down in a quiet, dimly lit place, close your eyes and concentrate on relaxing your whole body, starting with your toes and working your way up to the top of your head. Let each limb hang heavy in turn. Concentrate on breathing deeply, exhaling slowly with a slight sigh. Ten minutes of this a day will help you to feel calmer.

MEDITATION This is similar to relaxation, but is best done in a sitting position. Close your eyes, and go round the body trying to relax each part. Then, when you are feeling calmer, repeat a word or syllable over and over again, or count your breath, for between five and ten minutes. As thoughts come into your mind, let them pass through, and keep focusing on your word or the counting technique.

ANXIETY

Anxiety is basically a fear reaction. Faced with a difficult situation, it activates the adrenal glands to produce adrenaline, causing trembling, sweating and shallow, rapid breathing. The whole body is tense and jumpy. Anxiety is linked to panic attacks; if these occur in particular situations, they are known as situational anxiety states or phobias. A well-known phobia is *agoraphobia*, a fear of open spaces. Psychotherapy or behaviour therapy, where the patient is encouraged and supported gradually to confront her phobia, is effective in helping sufferers.

For milder forms of anxiety, try to stay as still as you can inside as the anxiety sweeps over you. Try to listen to your feelings and fears. Wait for the anxiety to pass, and continue to work on staying calm when it's over. This may be difficult to do at first, but with practice it should get easier and the anxiety attacks less frequent.

DEPRESSION

True depressive illness is more common in women than in men. This is not the same as the ups and downs in mood we all experience in our everyday lives; with real depression it is very hard, if not impossible, to get out of it without help. Depressives feel worthless and that life is meaningless. For women hormonal imbalances may contribute to depressive episodes, but many of the factors mentioned above can also lead to depression.

Medically, depression is divided into two categories: *endogenous depression*, which is caused by a chemical upset in the brain; and *exogenous* or *reactive depression*, which is caused by external factors, such as the death of a close family member or divorce. Manic depression, a severe form, occurs when the sufferer goes through periods of depression or mania (agitation, agression and wildness) or both.

A very depressed person may be withdrawn, uninterested in life, frequently untidy, apathetic and lethargic. They may also suffer from loss of appetite, lack of sex drive, and insomnia or a desire to stay in bed all the time.

TREATMENT Serious depression needs professional help. Your doctor may be able to arrange for a social or health worker to come and see you to talk over your problems. She may also prescribe sleeping pills and/or anti-depressants (effective for endogenous depression) or tranquillisers to get you over the worst. These are potentially addictive and should be used with caution. Withdrawal from such drugs can mimic depressive symptoms. However, it is more important to come to terms with the problem – drugs alone cannot solve anything, only dull the pain. Psychotherapy has helped many sufferers, although this can be expensive, especially as it requires a long-term commitment. Counselling is a particularly useful therapy for problem-solving, as the counsellor aims to help you find out what you think is wrong with your life and jointly work out ways of dealing with it. Other women have found joining a women's group or self-help group beneficial. Helplines such as the Samaritans offer an excellent listening service.

In very severe cases specialist psychiatric help or even hospital admission may be needed.

British Association for Counselling, 1 Regent Place, Rugby, Warwick-shire CV21 2PJ. Tel: 0788 578328/9.
Relate: National Marriage Guidance, Herbert Gray College, Little Church Street, Rugby CV21 3AP. Tel: 0788 573241.
Samaritans, 17 Uxbridge Road, Slough, Berkshire SL1 1SN. Look in your telephone directory for your local branch.

ANOREXIA AND BULIMIA NERVOSA

Anorexia nervosa Sometimes known as 'the slimmer's disease', anorexia nervosa is deliberate self-starvation. It affects about 1 in 500 young women, and is potentially fatal: it is possible literally to starve to death. Starvation takes its toll on the body, with periods stopping, constipation, hair loss and swelling. Anorexics are often highly active despite their low calorie intake, and commonly have a distorted body image. This is probably a symptom of the illness, as they cannot see how thin they are.

Bulimia nervosa This is more common because it is easier to hide. Often starting in the late teens, girls eat huge amounts of food, then purge themselves either by making themselves sick or using laxatives. Continued vomiting and diarrhoea can have a serious effect on the body: the throat and stomach can be injured, preventing essential nutrients from being absorbed, tooth decay sets in from vomited stomach acid, and vital vitamins and body salts are lost.

Both of these eating disorders are getting more common, even affecting girls as young as eight or nine. Men and boys suffer too, but nowhere near as often as girls.

Why should women use food like this?

Stress seems to be a key factor (see page 18). Poor eating habits result, adding more stress, and the woman is in a vicious downward spiral. Feelings of insecurity and a lack of self-esteem are also important psychological factors. Another theory is that the woman cannot cope with her life, but represses her feelings of frustration and anger. She feels she has no control – except over her own body. This can be coupled with a desire to remain childlike while still achieving the ideal of the thin woman.

Bulimia is more common in certain jobs, like dancing, modelling and gymnastics, where weight and performance are all-important. Being in control is essential; bulimics fear that once they start eating they won't be able to stop. To regain control, they purge their bodies.

Where to get help
The important thing is to get help soon. If you are suffering from either of these disorders, accepting that you have a problem and that you need help may be the most difficult thing you have to do.
SPECIAL CLINICS See your GP; she will know if there is a special clinic for eating disorders near you.
COUNSELLING This has helped many people for all sorts of problems, particularly to build self-esteem, and bring back a sense of control in their lives.

ALTERNATIVES FOR HEALTH

Many doctors these days accept that they don't have all the answers and welcome the growth of alternative medicine. Gone are the days of the rigid sceptic who took offence if you suggested anything other than orthodox medicine.

The five major therapies are chiropractic, osteopathy, homeopathy, herbalism and acupuncture. They all operate on a holistic principle, treating the whole person with a specific programme tailored to the individual's needs. The aim is to improve self-healing, and restore wholeness.

Chiropractic This deals particularly with mechanical disorders of the spine and pelvis such as lumbago, sciatica, neck pain, etc. It uses X-rays to help with treatment, which is a form of careful manipulation.

Osteopathy A well-known therapy which is widely available, it is similar to chiropractic and relies on manipulation of the musculo-skeletal system.

Backache is a very common problem for which conventional medicine has often very little to offer. Osteopaths and chiropracters have gained respect in the medical and lay world by offering some hope of relief. Both these therapies can also help with other conditions, including stress-related illnesses, arthritis and digestive problems.

Homeopathy This uses natural substances to effect a cure. Homeopathy is based on the principle that whatever causes the disease in large doses can in small doses cure it. Some of these remedies can be quite powerful, even interacting with conventional drugs. Care must be taken in pregnancy.

Herbalism Plants or plant extracts are used in herbal remedies. A herbalist looks for the root cause of the illness and the preparations aim to improve your general health. Other treatments using plants include aromatherapy, where essential oils from plants are diluted in a carrying oil and applied to the skin or added to baths; and Bach Flower Remedies, which work in a similar way to homeopathy, but address the emotional state of the patient rather than her physical symptoms.

Acupuncture An ancient Chinese method of treating illness and maintaining health, in which natural sources of energy within the body are regulated through the insertion of very fine needles into specific points on the body. It can also be used to induce anaesthesia. These points are carefully selected sites that correspond to organs or body functions. This stimulates a healing energy (Chi) which passes to the painful or diseased part of the body. Again the emphasis is on treating the person as a whole.

Other techniques becoming available include reflexology and shiatsu.

Reflexology This involves massage of the feet, which are said to have every organ of the body represented in a reflex zone. Massage of the zones can help to release tension. There is no anatomical backing to this theory, but some people find the massage very helpful.

Shiatsu Similarly to reflexology, Shiatsu works on the acupuncture points. Pressure is applied to the 'problem' points to change the energy relationships in the body. As in acupuncture and reflexology, the area treated may be far away from the original complaint.

COMMON HEALTH CONCERNS

THE SKIN

THE SUN AND SKINCARE

Ultraviolet rays from the sun damage the skin, making it less elastic, more fragile, yellowish and furrowed. The main cause of wrinkles is exposure to the sun. No amount of expensive creams will prevent you getting them; wearing a wide-brimmed hat in the sun is the best beauty treatment you can give your face.

If you want a sun tan, dermatological advice is to buy a fake tan cream and apply the colour directly. Better still, use one with a sunscreen incorporated into it.

Skin cancer (*melanoma*) is on the increase, and women most at risk are those with pale skins who freckle easily. If you must go out in the sun, make sure you know your skin type and use creams with higher protection factors if you are sensitive to the sun. Use creams with at least sun protection six or higher. Reapply sun cream after swimming, and watch the bits that catch the skin, such as ears, shoulders, nose and, if you are topless, nipples.

Babies should be kept out of the sun; don't let toddlers play in the sun without any clothes on, and use sunblocks on exposed areas of skin. Sunburn in childhood should be avoided at all costs, especially as it seems to increase the risks of skin trouble later on.

Any change in a mole or freckle should be reported to your doctor straight away: change in shape, looking irregular in shape or colour, bleeding or discharge, itching or looking inflamed.

SUNBEDS These are designed to shine a similar light to that of sunlight, and have the same aging effect on the skin. No one knows yet if they increase the risk of skin cancer. Probably best avoided.

CELLULITE AND FAT

There is no mystery about what cellulite is – it's fat. The name was invented to describe the stubborn, dimply fat that can appear on the body. Expensive treatments were then invented to get rid of it.

Fat on the hips and thighs, for example, is the last to be lost when you are dieting. Men don't seem to suffer as a rule, perhaps because they don't lay fat down in these areas so readily as women. There is no scientific evidence to suggest that cellulite is due to the accumulation of toxic products, and it's not a disease. It will disappear eventually if you pay particular attention to exercising these areas.

TREATMENTS These range from massages and creams to muscle toning stimulators. They certainly make you more aware of your body, and are generally relaxing and enjoyable, but as far as dissolving away cellulite goes, I'm afraid the results are disappointing. The magic ingredients in the creams just can't penetrate the skin layer and get to the fat. Massage may increase blood circulation and lymph drainage, but that doesn't break up fat cells more quickly. A brisk walk would do more for your muscles than the weak, electrically induced contractions given in toning treatments. Bust firming treatments are no better.

You can spend a lot of money on these 'cures', but their only value will be if they make you feel good and heighten your awareness of your body. A work out in an exercise class followed by a swim and a sauna would be cheaper and better for you.

DIGESTIVE PROBLEMS

Fortunately, women seem to be protected from some stomach troubles, like peptic ulcers, by their hormones. (Peptic ulcers are more common in men, although women lose their protection after the menopause.) However, women are more prone to gall-stones and irritable bowel syndrome (see below).

GALL-STONES (Cholelithiasis)

The typical sufferer of gall-stones is fair, fat, fertile and forty (not very scientific but easy to remember!).

The gall bladder sits under the liver on the upper right side of the abdomen. Gall-stones come mainly from too much cholesterol in a fatty diet. Many remain 'silent' and produce no symptoms at all. If this is the case, and it is discovered by chance that you do have gall-stones, fatty foods should be avoided. Fibre also helps to keep cholesterol levels down, so plenty of roughage should be eaten. If you're overweight, try to lose those extra pounds. If, however, a gall-stone gets stuck in the neck of the gall bladder trouble follows. The gall bladder stores bile before it drains into the small bowel. If the way out is blocked, inflammation of the gall bladder (*cholecystitis*) can occur, with right-sided abdominal pain, temperature, nausea and maybe vomiting. Jaundice may suggest the bile drainage is blocked.

TREATMENT Antibiotics usually settle things down, but if problems continue removal of the gall bladder (*cholcystectomy*) may be a good idea. In the past this was a full-scale abdominal operation. These days a new technique of removing the gall bladder through a *laparoscope* (page 47) has been developed. There is no big incision, and it involves only a short stay in hospital.

IRRITABLE BOWEL SYNDROME

As many as fifteen in every hundred people have irritable bowel syndrome, and ten of them will be women. It can be difficult to diagnose as the symptoms are all similar to other problems, but the trouble is usually a combination of abdominal pain, a feeling of bloating or wind, and difficulties with constipation or diarrhoea.

There are many theories about the cause; it could be diet, constipation, food allergy or intolerance, stress or a combination of these.

TREATMENT Try to understand your own body and what upsets it, anything from food to stress or anxiety. Avoid triggering factors. Your doctor will be able to help with bowel-relaxing drugs (e.g. Colofac).

British Digestive Foundation, 3 St. Andrew's Place, London NW1 4LB. Tel: 071-486 0341.

CIRCULATORY PROBLEMS

VARICOSE VEINS

These are very common in both men and women, but women tend to make more fuss about them because their legs are on show. Varicose veins seem to run in families, inheriting a weakness in the veins so that they don't empty properly and stay full of blood. Straining to pass a motion can make things worse. Pregnancy also puts an increased back pressure on the veins.

Varicose veins can be quite uncomfortable, making your legs ache, especially if you have been standing for any length of time, or at the end of the day. Support tights or stockings can give relief throughout the day. You can get these from the chemist or sometimes on prescription.

TREATMENT Options are injecting the veins to make the vein walls stick together (usually done in the clinic) or having the vein stripped out, which requires a stay in hospital.

PILES (Haemorrhoids)

Piles are varicose veins of the anal area and are very common in pregnancy. This is not a serious condition but it can be very uncomfortable. You should always consult your doctor if you suspect piles.

Internal piles These cause bleeding (bright red) during a bowel motion and can sometimes come out (prolapse), causing a feeling of heaviness. There may also be a discharge of mucoid material, itching and constipation.

External Piles These are visible on the anal surface – they can look like a bunch of grapes, and may become swollen and tender if a clot forms.

If you have piles and find it difficult to keep your bottom clean and comfortable, try using moistened baby wipes or cotton wool instead of or as well as toilet paper.

TREATMENT Various treatments are available: injections to shrivel the piles, stretching the anus under an anaesthetic or surgically removing the piles. Eat plenty of fibre to keep out of trouble with constipation and excessive straining.

Bleeding from the back passage is not normal: tell your doctor.

MIGRAINE

Migraine affects more women than men. No one knows why this should be, but it is known that a tendency to get migraine can be inherited. Research has looked at various chemicals in food and drink without coming up with a theory about migraine in general.

An attack is usually a painful throbbing headache, often over one eye, preceded by visual disturbances such as flashing lights and zig zag lines. There is sometimes nausea and vomiting, and sometimes numbness down one side of the body.

Some women find that they react to food containing tyramine, such as cheese or chocolate, or to low blood sugar levels when meals are missed (if this is the case, make a point of having regular meals).

Stress can set off an attack, but it's often when the stress is over that the migraine strikes.

TREATMENT First, your blood pressure needs to be checked. If it's high it may be making things worse. If you have a migraine attack for the first time when you're on the Pill you should stop it immediately (and use another form of contraception).

Simple analgesics, like paracetamol or aspirin, can relieve the headache pain. Lying down in a darkened room also helps most sufferers. The herbal remedy feverfew has been shown to reduce the number of migraine attacks, but this is not available on prescription and the quality of preparations you can buy is very variable. If the migraine continues to be a problem, upsetting your daily life, preventative measures are available. Beta-blocking drugs act against the chemical serotonin (one of the agents thought to be responsible for migraine).

Some women seem to get attacks related to their menstrual cycle. This may be due to low oestrogen levels just before and during periods. Oestradiol given under the skin before and during menstruation has already had very good results.

British Migraine Association, 178a High Road, Byfleet, Weybridge, Surrey KT14 7ED. Tel: 0932 352468.

RAYNAUD'S DISEASE

'Cold hands, warm heart', so the saying goes, but cold hands can mean a miserable life for women with Raynaud's disease. As many as one in five people have it to some degree, more women than men. The circulation in the body's extremities goes into spasm, affecting the fingers, toes, ears or nose. Tissue damage can occur in severe cases. With exposure to the cold, first pins and needles are experienced in the fingers, then they go deathly white. As the fingers heat up they then turn bluish and red.

TREATMENT Mainly self-help: avoid the cold and take special care to keep your hands and feet warm.

Recent research has shown that oestrogen increases the likelihood of vessel spasm, while progesterone relaxes the vessels. This may provide some clue to hormonal treatment in the future.

Raynauds and Scleroderma Association Trust, 112 Crewe Road, Alsager, Cheshire ST7 2JA. Tel: 0270-872776.

URINARY PROBLEMS

CYSTITIS

Cystitis actually means inflammation of the bladder and for some women can be a recurring problem.

A typical attack starts with you needing to urinate more frequently, just passing a little urine each time, and it starts to hurt especially at the end of the stream; your lower abdomen may feel tender, the urine may change to a cloudy colour or even be blood stained. It can be very uncomfortable. Why it happens and to certain women isn't clearly understood. One reason may be that the urethra, which drains the urine from the bladder, is very short compared with the long urethra in men and is positioned between the clitoris and the vagina. It is therefore easy for bacteria to travel up to the bladder. If you don't sit down completely to pass urine you're in danger of leaving some in the bladder. This could get infected and set off another attack of cystitis. Don't perch above the toilet even in a public convenience: sit down and make sure your bladder is empty.

Sexual activity can also send bacteria up into the bladder.

Only half of women with cystitis actually have bacteria growing in their urine, which means not all cystitis episodes need to be treated with antibiotics. *Urethral syndrome* is the name given to cystitis when there is no infection.

How to avoid urethral syndrome

First of all, make sure there isn't any local infection that is being sent up into the bladder – think about thrush (page 86), chlamydia (page 87) or trichomoniasis (page 87) infections in the vagina. Do you have a discharge of any kind?

Some women are allergic to soap, bubble bath or washing powder. Sexual intercourse, however, is probably a prime factor.

To minimise the risk of urethral syndrome follow these guidelines. To ensure good hygiene, take a bath or shower before making love. If your vagina gets dry, use a lubricant (KY jelly) to help keep things smooth. Ideally drink a litre/1¾ pints of fluid before intercourse and get up and empty your bladder afterwards; some women find washing their vulva after sex helps too. Discourage your partner from exploring the area around the anus. Try different positions for intercourse.

In the menopause the vagina gets drier and the skin in the area gets thinner and weaker; inflammation is more common. Hormone replacement therapy or local oestrogen cream may be necessary here.

Pregnancy makes the muscle wall of the ureter, which drains the urine from the kidneys to the bladder, relax and the urine gets stagnant. Infection can start and can be quite serious if not treated.

TREATMENT Drink, drink and drink again. Take two paracetamol tablets, and go to bed with a hot water bottle. Give this time to work (e.g. twelve to twenty-four hours), but if things are getting worse – pain, frequency, blood in the urine – you must seek help from your doctor. You will need to give a specimen of urine taken in the middle of the stream (MSU) into a sterile container. Antibiotics are usually prescribed. If this is a continuing problem then low-dose antibiotics taken for a length of time may be considered.

WELL-WOMAN SCREENING

Well-woman clinics are being set up in some forward-thinking family practices to provide screening checks on a regular basis. These should include a blood pressure check, a breast examination, cervical smear and internal pelvic examination. At the moment, the advice is to have a

FEMALE PELVIC ORGANS

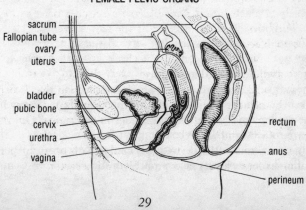

sacrum
Fallopian tube
ovary
uterus
bladder
pubic bone
cervix
urethra
vagina
rectum
anus
perineum

cervical smear every three to five years. A well-organised family planning clinic can also do this for you even if you don't need contraception – ring and check first.

Warning signs like changes in your bleeding pattern, bleeding after intercourse or between your periods may all mean something is not quite right. Potential problems picked up early can be sorted out quickly. Find out what symptoms you should look for on page 37; if you're worried about anything don't delay, visit your doctor. These days more and more women are training to be doctors. Over the last ten years the number of female GPs has increased by over 75 per cent. It's likely, therefore, that your practice will include a female doctor, which is very reassuring for those women who find it hard to discuss the ins and outs of periods and discharges with a man. In this book I've referred to doctors as female for a change.

VULVA

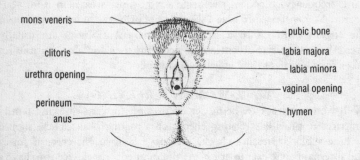

mons veneris — pubic bone
clitoris — labia majora
— labia minora
urethra opening —
— vaginal opening
perineum —
anus — — hymen

CERVICAL SMEAR
The best advice is to start having cervical smears as soon as you start having sex. Some girls combine a check up with a visit to discuss contraception. From then on repeat it every three to five years until you reach seventy.

Having a smear test is simple and painless. It is best done when you're not having a period. You need to lie down, usually on your back with your knees bent and relaxed outwards. (Some doctors do this with you lying on your left side with your knees bent up.) To put you at ease, the doctor normally covers you from the waist down to mid thigh

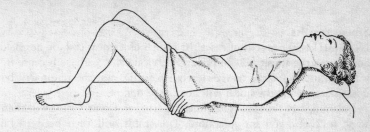

with a cloth. The lips of the vulva are opened and a speculum (a beak-like device that opens inside you), which has been lubricated with a little jelly, is put into the vagina. Once the cervix is in view it's gently wiped with a wooden spatula; this doesn't hurt, perhaps a slight scraping feeling, nothing more. The cells that come off are put on a slide and rapidly put in a fixing solution. The cells are studied later under the microscope. When you have this test your doctor can also study the cervix, looking for polyps (page 57), cervical erosion or cervicitis (see below).

SPECULUM EXAMINATION

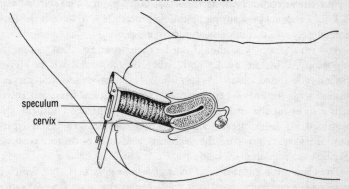

speculum
cervix

Cervical erosion This is absolutely normal and very common. It means that the inside layer of cells lining the cervix actually get turned inside out, making the cervix look red. This change in the cervix is under hormonal control – erosions are common in pregnancy and whilst on the Pill, uncommon after the menopause. No treatment is necessary unless you have a troublesome discharge – the glandular cells can be frozen off (*cryosurgery*) or burnt off (*diathermy* or *cautery*).

Cervicitis This is an inflamed cervix, but some women have a reddened cervix without any evidence of infection. If your smear is negative and infection swabs are clear, then there is nothing to worry about.

Smear results

NORMAL In 90 per cent of cases the results of a smear test are normal. Sometimes the smear fails to pick up cervical cells, perhaps because it was difficult to see the cervix clearly. In such cases, the result will be unsatisfactory and the smear will need to be done again.

Inflammatory cells are sometimes reported and your doctor will then want to check you for infection. The smear will then need to be repeated in a year.

ABNORMAL This is known as *dyskaryosis*, and it is graded in terms of severity. The cell picture changes (with progressively bigger nuclei in the middle of the cells) the more severe the abnormality. Sometimes the smear will report cells suggesting a wart virus infection (*human papilloma virus*).

POSITIVE In a very small number of cases the smear shows cells suggesting invasive cancer of the cervix. Usually further tests, like a biopsy, are necessary to confirm the diagnosis.

If your smear comes back as abnormal don't panic. You will be asked back for a *colposcopy* – a simple, painless procedure – to look at the cervix more closely and sort out any abnormal areas.

As with a smear, you should not be menstruating when you go for a colposcopy. You are awake and either lie on your back or sit in a specially designed chair. A speculum is inserted and the cervix is studied with the aid of a colposcope – an instrument like a microscope with a light on the end. Mild acetic acid is painted on and the effect examined. If some areas look abnormal samples are taken (this is sometimes enough to cure the problem), and laser or cautery treatment may be required later (see below).

The usual problem is *cervical intraepithelial neoplasia* (CIN), which has replaced the old name dysplasia, graded in increasing abnormality from CIN 1 to CIN 3. This is not cancer because the abnormalities are confined to the surface layer and have not invaded through to deeper tissue. However, if the abnormal areas were left they might go on to form cancer after many years. Wart virus changes on the cervix are also treated in the same way; they, too, may be linked to cancer developing later on.

TREATMENT The aim is to destroy the cells, either by removing them with a hot loop or vaporising them with a laser. This is done while you are awake. Local anaesthetic is either injected or spread as a gel on to the cervix first. The treatment itself can sometimes be a bit uncomfortable, but there should be a reassuring nurse with you to hold your hand if you're nervous. Take a friend with you for additional support. Some units have a television screen so you can watch your cervix on the box, if you feel like it. You will need to rest afterwards, so make sure you have a clear day. Ensure you've got sanitary pads at home.

Once you've had the treatment you may be asked to come and have a follow-up colposcopy or smear in a few months in case you need more treatment. If you get the all clear, you will only need cervical smears once a year.

Don't be depressed if CIN happens to you: it's very common, it's easy to treat and you may well have avoided bigger problems in the future. Try not to let it affect your sex life, and get yourself fitted with a diaphragm if it makes you feel better — the cervix certainly appreciates the protection. Ask in the colposcopy clinic about sex after treatment — it is usually all right after the next period (which is often heavier than normal).

If you've had an abnormal smear and a colposcopy you can reduce the risk of further problems:
- limit your number of sexual partners
- use a diaphragm for contraception
- use a condom if in doubt about your partner's past
- stop smoking
- have regular smears.

> *I had a smear in June 1990. I got a letter in January 1991 saying I had to go back for another. I phoned the surgery straight away and asked them why there was no explanation of why I should go back. The receptionist gave the result of the first smear over the phone, she said there were abnormal cells on the smear. They had left it for six months to tell me because I had been suffering from thrush on and off and they had to make sure that wasn't the cause of it.*
>
> *The results from the second smear showed that the cells had progressed since the last smear. The doctor said there was nothing to worry about, it didn't necessarily mean cancer. He sent me to Southmead Hospital for possible laser treatment.*
>
> *I went in February. The gynae-consultant showed me on the t.v. the area which needed to be removed, saying it was only the size of a match head. He didn't use laser treatment, but removed the area and the tissue around it there and then. It didn't hurt. He was*

very nice and explained everything to me. I was in and out in ten minutes. I had another smear after that, and the results were OK. Then you have to go back a year later – I'm going in September, for a check up.

PELVIC EXAMINATION

After your smear the doctor will examine you with her hands. Wearing a clean plastic glove, she will put two fingers gently into the vagina up to the cervix. The other hand will be on your lower abdomen. With a rocking movement she will be able to feel the shape and position of your uterus, and any enlargement or tenderness in the tubes or ovaries.

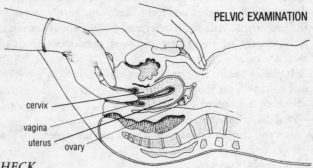

PELVIC EXAMINATION

cervix

vagina

uterus

ovary

BREAST CHECK

All women worry about breast cancer, and it is now the second most common cause of death among women in Britain after heart disease. Breast cancer killed about 13,000 women in the UK in 1990 alone.

As more than 90 per cent of breast cancers are detected by women themselves, I believe it is essential that each woman be aware of her breasts and their normal cyclical changes. Although the effectiveness of a formal breast self-examination at a set time each month has been questioned, for some women it provides a useful ritual, and you should do whatever works best for you. If you don't want a routine, just soap yourself without a flannel when you wash, feeling the breasts and under the armpits. Remember, breast cancer in women under forty is very rare, and four out of five breast lumps are benign. After the age of forty, the risk of breast cancer steadily increases (page 178).

Breast self-examination

It's best to examine your breasts just after your period; if you're in the menopause set a specific time aside, perhaps on the first day of each

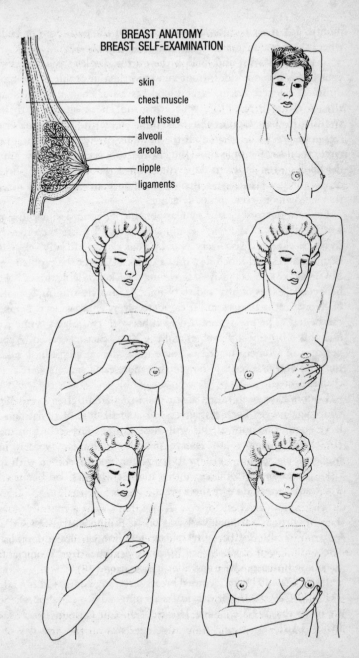

BREAST ANATOMY
BREAST SELF-EXAMINATION

skin
chest muscle
fatty tissue
alveoli
areola
nipple
ligaments

month. It's most comfortable to do this in the bathroom or bedroom where there is a mirror, before taking a bath or shower.

Strip to the waist and look in the mirror. Look at your breasts with your hands by your sides, front view and then in profile. Check for any dimples, puckered skin, large blood vessels or change in the shape or size of either breast. Lift your arms and check again. Is there any swelling in the armpit or above the breast? Next, in the shower or bath, feel your breasts all over with the flat part of your hand – it's best to circle round the nipple from the outside in – feeling for any lumps or thickening. It's easier to do if your skin is wet and soapy. Check the nipple for any discharge, a little crust is normal, but a heavy discharge that's brown or green or bloody is not.

Let your doctor know as soon as possible if you find something you're worried about. If you don't examine your own breasts then they ought to be checked at least every year by your doctor. Ideally, any clinical examination should include a breast check whatever the problem.

MAMMOGRAPHY This is a screening check available for all women between the ages of fifty and sixty-four. It involves shining a small dose of X-ray on the breasts and it can detect very small cancers before they can be felt. The breasts are squeezed between two plates (some women find this a bit uncomfortable) and the X-ray pictures taken. About 70 per cent of women invited to come for a mammogram have taken up the offer and first results showed that more early cancers were detected than expected.

Doubts have been raised about making mammograms available to a wider age range. Each test gives you a small dose of radiation, and a large enough amount of this will cause cancer. The feeling in medical circles is, therefore, to reserve mammography for women in the high-risk age group, i.e. fifty to sixty-four, and to women with special risks, for example, someone with a mother who has had breast cancer. The test is repeated every three years.

The Women's National Cancer Control Campaign (WNCCC). Tel: 071-729 2229. Offers a telephone helpline on cervical and breast screening. Open 9.30 am – 4.30 pm every weekday. Women trained in counselling can advise and offer information.
Tel: 071-729 4915 for recorded breast screening advice (24 hours).
Tel: 071-729 5061 for cervical screening advice (24 hours). Send a s.a.e. to the WNCC, Suna House, 128–130 Curtain Road, London EC2A 3AR.

BACUP is a cancer information and support organisation and offers information over the phone (free when calling from outside London, tel: 0800 181199, and local rate charge when calling from inner London, tel: 071-608 1661). It also provides a counselling service face-to-face, at present available only in London. Tel: 071-608 1038.

GENERAL HEALTH

Have your blood pressure checked. This needs to be done every five years, and more frequently if you're on the Pill or hormone replacement therapy. If you have a problem, keep your blood pressure down by losing weight, cutting down on your salt intake, and taking up yoga or some relaxation therapy. If your blood pressure stays high, you will probably benefit from drug therapy which cuts down the risk of a heart attack or stroke occurring in the future.

Some clinics do a cholesterol and lipids screen, ask if this is necessary for you. If someone in your family has had circulatory trouble or a heart attack at an unusually young age you may be at risk.

Have your weight checked and discuss it if it's a problem.

Check your alcohol intake – it should be no more than 14 units a week (1 unit = 1 glass of wine, 300 ml/½ pint of beer or cider, 1 measure spirits).

If you smoke, get help to give up.

WARNING SIGNS – WHAT TO LOOK FOR

The sooner you realise that something is not right the sooner it can be sorted out. The following symptoms should be reported promptly to your doctor. Not all of them mean that there is anything serious, but it's best to be on the safe side.

General

Feeling excessively tired: *anaemia, stress (page 18)*. Are you off your food and losing weight?: *stomach and bowel disorders, serious general illness*
Persistent cough or coughing up blood: *chronic chest infection, lung cancer*
Lumps in your abdomen: *cysts or tumours of the ovary (page 61), bowel etc, hernia, fibroids (page 56), stomach or bowel growths*
Pain in the upper abdomen: *gall-stones (page 25), hiatus hernia, stomach ulcer*
Pain in the lower abdomen: *irritable bowel syndrome (page 25), pelvic inflammation (page 59), twisting or bleeding ovarian cyst (page 61), colitis, diverticulitis*

Skin

Moles – changing shape, bleeding or discharging, itchy or inflamed: *sun-related change, skin cancer (page 23)*

Reproductive system

Bleeding or spotting after intercourse/between your periods: *cervical erosion (page 31) or polyps (page 57), Pill problems (page 64), cervical CIN and cancer (page 32), pelvic infection*

Heavier periods: *hormone disturbance (page 49), fibroids (page 56), endometriosis (page 57), IUD (page 68), stress (page 18)*

Absent or scanty periods: *normal pattern, pregnancy (page 100), stress (page 18), polycystic ovaries (page 61), premature menopause (page 163)*

Painful periods: *normal pattern, endometriosis (page 57), chronic pelvic infection (page 59), IUD (page 68)*

Pain with intercourse: *endometriosis (page 57), chronic pelvic infection (page 68), vaginal infection (page 85), poor lubrication (page 165)*

Bleeding after the menopause (one year without periods): *dry vagina, endometrial polyps (page 57), endometrial cancer (page 61)*

Vaginal discharge: *thrush (page 87), trichomoniasis (page 87), chlamydia (page 87), gonorrhoea (page 88), Pill (page 64), IUD (page 68), cervical erosion (page 31) or polyps (page 57), pregnancy (page 100)*

Breasts

Tingling, fullness, discomfort: *pre-menstrual changes, early pregnancy, breastfeeding*

Lumps in the breasts or armpits: *cysts, fibroadenosis, tumours (page 178), breast abscess*

Nipple discharge: *breast infection, tumours (page 178)*

Altered breast appearance, nipple pulled in, dimpled skin: *tumour, malignant growth (page 178)*

Bowels and bladder

Upset bowel routine: *diet changes, irritable bowel syndrome (page 25), colitis, diverticulitis, bowel cancer*

Blood in the motion: *piles (page 26), colitis, bowel cancer*

Blood in the urine: *cystitis (page 28), bladder tumour*

Pain on passing urine: *cystitis (page 28), vaginal infection (page 85)*

Incontinence of urine: *infection, pelvic floor weakness/stress (page 174), nervous bladder/urgency (page 174), pregnancy (page 100)*

—2—

HORMONES AND THE

REPRODUCTIVE

SYSTEM

At times of key change in women's lives – when they begin their periods, in pregnancy, when they reach the menopause – the levels of sex hormones in their bodies change too. It is these changes that are to blame for the physical, and probably many of the emotional, discomforts women experience at these times. During their reproductive years, women have consistently high levels of sex hormones which fluctuate each month to determine ovulation and menstruation. It is this constant fluctuation that probably makes some women difficult to live with at the end of each menstrual cycle (although it may simply be that they are super sensitive to these hormones), contributes to post-natal depression, and makes some women feel very sexy around ovulation.

What is a hormone?
A hormone is a very, very small protein messenger that travels round in the bloodstream with a job to do. Hormones come from various glands: the pituitary gland in the brain, the adrenal gland and the ovary. The female reproductive system depends on a complicated interlinking of hormones, each related to each other.

The part of the brain called the *hypothalamus* gives out the instructions. When your *oestrogen* level is low just after a period, the hypothalamus tells the pituitary gland (by producing a *gonadotrophin releasing hormone*, GnRH) to produce *follicle stimulating hormone* (FSH) in order to grow a new egg in the ovary and produce some more oestrogen. The uterus grows its lining again and at the right time the pituitary sends out what is known as a *luteinising hormone* (LH) to make you ovulate. The empty follicle that's left (the *corpus luteum*) is very good at producing *progesterone* and does so in the second half of the cycle (the luteal phase). This makes the pituitary stop sending out hormones. When the corpus luteum can't produce any more progesterone, the lining of the uterus collapses and menstruation occurs. At this point, oestrogen and progesterone are low again, so signals go to the brain to start the whole process again.

If, on the other hand, the egg is fertilised it will soon produce another hormone (*human chorionic gonadotrophin*, HCG), which tells the corpus luteum to carry on producing progesterone. HCG is the hormone measured in pregnancy tests.

Can hormones cause hairiness?

It is quite normal for women to have hair on their bodies, including on the abdomen and around the nipples. Excessive hairiness, however, may be due to a hormonal imbalance. If you're worried, see your doctor, who can check your hormone levels.

The adrenal gland and the ovary produce male-type hormones and their secretion can be increased in certain conditions. The most common is *polycystic ovarian syndrome*: ovulation doesn't work properly, there may be difficulties in getting pregnant, the ovaries look cystic, periods become irregular, you sometimes put on weight and get hairier.

More often no actual cause is found and the reason put down to an increased sensitivity to the androgen hormones produced in the ovary.
TREATMENT It's quite difficult to treat, with a wait of six to twelve months before any improvement. The combined Pill is worth a try, so is cyproterone acetate, an anti-androgen drug, combined with oestrogen.

Bleaching can make body hair much less noticeable, and electrolysis in expert hands gives a permanent result. This is suitable for facial hair.

Hormones and fatness

On the whole women are fatter than men (at forty, 16 per cent of women and 12 per cent of men are overweight). At puberty the hormone oestrogen decides where fat should be deposited – on the breasts and on the hips and thighs. So our hormones dictate where the fat should go, but they don't make us overweight.
THE PILL Taking the contraceptive Pill can cause an increase in appetite (progestogen) and some fluid retention (oestrogen), sometimes with a noticeable increase in weight. Many progestogen compounds (Primulot, Duphaston) tend to make you put on weight.

THE THYROID The hormones produced by the thyroid help to control our metabolic rate and weight balance. An underactive thyroid will slow us down mentally and physically; weight gain is another side-effect. Too much of the thyroid hormone *thyroxine* and our metabolism speeds up and the weight falls off. Thyroxine has been used for slimming, but has serious side-effects on the heart and nervous system.

MENSTRUAL DISORDERS

PREMENSTRUAL SYNDROME (PMS)

Almost all women know when their next period is due from how they feel. The most common symptoms at this time are feeling bloated and irritable. Many women put on weight, have a craving for carbohydrates or anything sweet, and feel generally depressed. They may suffer from headaches and backache, find it hard to concentrate, and their breasts may become bigger and tender. The hormone that has been blamed for

THE MENSTRUAL CYCLE

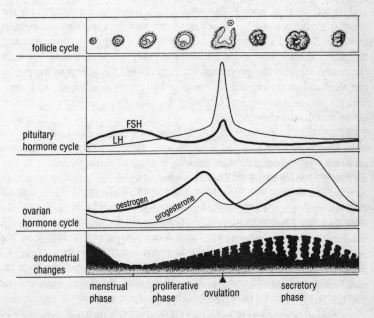

PMS is progesterone, which is the dominant hormone in the second half of the cycle. Certainly, progesterone affects the small muscles in the blood vessels and so more fluid appears in the circulation. It also relaxes the muscle in the bowel so that its contents are delayed. This means that loops of bowel are sitting around doing little with lots of gas in them. As a result, your clothes feel tight; some women even reserve skirts and trousers specially for the premenstrual week.

About one in twenty women are actually disabled by PMS and seek medical help. They find life very difficult in the premenstrual days – work, relationships and homelife all suffer.

Treatment of PMS

The good news is that in most cases of PMS there is nothing actually wrong with the body. It is now thought that some women are just more sensitive to oestrogen and progesterone. Unfortunately, this means that PMS can be difficult to treat. If you suspect you are suffering from PMS, first make a list of your symptoms in your diary, giving them marks out of ten if they change in severity. Keep this for three months to see if a pattern emerges.

The way to deal with PMS is mainly by self-help measures. Use the diary of symptoms to try to predict next month when the bad time is going to be, and if possible take measures to help you cope. Arrange stressful events – the in-laws coming to stay, or a confrontation with the boss – to miss the premenstrual days. If PMS is going to happen at the weekend, warn the family, prepare the meals in advance, and don't embark on full-scale spring cleaning. In addition, consider one or more of the activities below.

RELAXATION Some women find relaxation exercises and yoga classes help them generally to cope with the difficult days. To be most effective, these should be done regularly, not just during PMS.

EVENING PRIMROSE OIL This is a very interesting substance, rich in *gammalinolenic acid* (GLA), which has been commercially marketed for the treatment of PMS. Research suggests that PMS sufferers are deficient in GLA. This is an essential fatty acid, important in producing tissue hormones like *prostaglandins* (page 44). (GLA in the body is made from another essential fatty acid, cis-linolenic acid.) However, high adrenaline levels, cholesterol, viral infections, alcohol, and being short of zinc, magnesium or vitamin B6 can all slow up the production of GLA in the body.

Increasing your dietary intake of GLA is said to sort out the defect in your metabolism. Commercial preparations of evening primrose oil (Efamol, Efamast) contain both GLA and Vitamin E. The recommended dose is four capsules (40 mg each) twice a day. Efamast is now available on prescription for women with breast pain. You need to take evening primrose oil for as long as eight to twelve weeks before you can expect any improvement in your breasts. Research has still not convincingly proved any benefit from evening primrose oil over a placebo in the treatment of premenstrual syndrome and further trials are necessary.

In addition, increase your intake of GLA by eating oats, barley, black and red currants, gooseberries and borage oil. It's probably useful to take a vitamin supplement of Vitamin B6, too.

DRUGS Doctors have been confused for years about whether certain drugs do any good at all. Natural progesterone, for example, has been prescribed, but in certain trials some of the women who were given a placebo instead still got better. Many women find changing their diet and taking supplements are just as effective. Water tablets (Diamox) have been shown to help, as have oestrogens, and anti-inflammatory drugs (Ponstan), danazol (Danol) and buserilin (Suprefact). Buserilin is taken as a nasal spray and acts by switching off the pituitary so it can't stimulate the ovary. No hormones are produced so no periods arrive. It's very effective, but because it acts like the menopause, you can't stay on it for long as your bones will start to weaken. Danazol stops your periods as well; it can work very well, but many women put on weight, some get spotty and some have increased facial hair. The contraceptive Pill may be a less drastic way of coping with PMS if you need birth control as well.

PREGNANCY This is marvellous for most PMS sufferers as your hormones are on a plateau and you feel stable and predictable, although it is a rather drastic cure! The menopause has these advantages as well – something to look forward to.

ABSENCE OF PERIODS (*Amenorrhea*)

There are two types of *amenorrhea* – *primary*, which means never having had a period, and *secondary*, which means loss of periods in a women who has already begun to menstruate. Primary amenorrhea can run in families, or may be due to underweight, but should be investigated in girls of fourteen who have not developed normally (no breasts or pubic hair) and in girls of sixteen who have developed normally but have still not started their periods.

Secondary amenorrhea is normal in pregnancy, but stress, anorexia, hormonal imbalances, absence of ovulation, and chronic illnesses such as thyroid disease, anaemia and tuberculosis can also cause this.

TREATMENT See your doctor if amenorrhea lasts for more than six months; she may need to refer you to a specialist.

PAINFUL PERIODS (Dysmenorrhoea)

Dysmenorrhoea (literally meaning painful monthly loss) makes life difficult for 50 per cent of women aged between fifteen and twenty-five. It accounts for lots of time off work – in America alone 140 million hours a year.

Some women are quite disabled for two or three days a month with low abdominal cramp-like pain. The pain can be in the back or radiate down the thighs, and sometimes there is diarrhoea and vomiting as well. It is very difficult to carry on doing anything in this state.

Why do some women get painful periods?

Frustratingly, no one really knows, although a large number of women who have painful periods also have high levels of prostaglandins at the time of menstruation. On the positive side, however, it is possible to do something about the pain (see opposite).

Prostaglandins In most cases there is nothing wrong with the pelvis. (Painful periods seem to happen in cycles where an egg is produced – ovulatory cycles – which explains why the first few periods, when things are getting established, are usually painfree.) The pain may be due to high levels of prostaglandins (hormones that act locally) in the uterus. This in turn causes the uterine muscle to go into spasm, pinching off the blood supply. It is this that causes the cramp-like pain that comes and goes. Why some women should have these high levels of prostaglandins in the uterus isn't known.

Vasopressin A pituitary hormone that regulates water balance, *vasopressin*, can also cause uterine spasm. It too is increased in women who suffer period pain. Again, the reason is a mystery.

Pelvic inflammatory disease or endometriosis These can both make your periods painful and often heavy as well. If you suffer from increasing pain go and see your doctor (pages 57 and 59).

Help required!

The Greeks used dried snake and calf's gall, the Victorians tried leeches on the cervix – we've moved on a long way since then. For many women going to bed with some simple painkillers and a hot-water bottle while the pain is at its worst does the trick. Masturbation can also help to relieve the spasm.

DRUGS Anti-inflammatory drugs (Ponstan and Indocid) reduce the production of the uterine-cramping prostaglandins, and help four out of five women. They can also reduce the amount of flow and shorten the period. Take the tablets as soon as the bleeding starts for the two to three days that your period is painful. Don't take them on an empty stomach, as they can be very irritating to the stomach lining.

THE PILL Another way of reducing the pain is to stop ovulation by taking the Pill. This suits some women (page 64).

ALTERNATIVE MEASURES In desperation some women have looked to alternative medicine for relief. Acupuncture (page 23), homeopathy (page 22) and aromatherapy (page 22) can help. In some cases conventional medicine can't solve the problem.

PREGNANCY The really drastic solution for some women is to have a baby – afterwards the pain improves dramatically or disappears. Doctors wondered if it was the cervix stretching that improved things, but operations to open (dilate) the cervix gently in sufferers were a resounding failure. It is possible that the nerve networks in the uterus are so stretched by pregnancy and labour that sensation is diminished in this area afterwards.

PELVIC PAIN

Many women get bouts of pelvic pain now and then. Some find it really gets them down and begins to interfere with their daily life. The pain can be a period-type cramping pain, coming and going, or a constant dull ache. Some women feel a dragging sensation which is worse at period times. If you have pain ask yourself some questions.

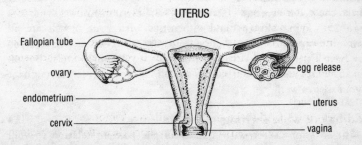

UTERUS

Fallopian tube — ovary — endometrium — cervix — egg release — uterus — vagina

Is the pain related to your periods or ovulation in the middle of the month?

Ovulation Pain experienced at ovulation is a mixed blessing – it may be uncomfortable, but at least it is a sign that everything is in working order. Ovulation occurs two weeks before your next period, which in a four-week cycle comes halfway between periods. Any discomfort is usually felt on one side or the other of the lower abdomen and only lasts a few hours. The pain can be stabbing, but it is more usually a dull ache. This is due to the follicle in the ovary stretching and then bursting to release the egg and surrounding fluid.

Periods Dysmenorrhoea isn't usually a symptom of disease (page 44), but for the older woman it may mean problems with pelvic inflammatory disease (page 59), endometriosis (page 57), or fibroids (page 56). In such cases, the pain usually starts a few days before the period and builds up to a peak during the first two or three days.

Does intercourse make the pain worse?

Endometriosis/Pelvic inflammatory disease If the ovaries, tubes and uterus are not very mobile due to scar formation they will not normally move with the thrusting penis during intercourse. The ovaries may be stuck down near the top of the vagina and will obviously be pushed during sex – this can be quite sore. Endometriosis and chronic pelvic inflammatory disease can cause this.

Congested Veins Some women have big, congested veins in their pelvis, for what reason we don't know. This can be uncomfortable, especially when standing and at the end of the day, and during intercourse. Drugs to stop ovulation help (Depo-Provera), and some women have found relief with relaxation techniques.

Are your bowels okay?

Irritable bowel syndrome Bowel upset is the most common cause of pain in the pelvic area and is sometimes called irritable bowel syndrome (page 25). Pain, bloating and difficulties with your bowels are all common symptoms. There can be diarrhoea, or constipation, and you may have little warning that you need to open your bowels. Bowel-relaxing drugs are available but it's a good idea to increase the roughage in your diet as well.

Finding out what's wrong

A visit to your doctor with a diary of the pain in relation to your periods, bowel movements and intercourse will be very helpful in making a correct diagnosis. It is also a useful checklist for you on the day. Think if anything in particular makes the pain worse or makes it better, and note this down too.

At the doctor's you will probably be given a pelvic examination (page 34), which should show up any problem with tenderness in the pelvic area. The uterus will be checked to see if it moves normally, and the ovaries individually felt to see if they are tender.

LAPAROSCOPY If anything suggests there is a problem, the doctor will arrange for you to be seen by a specialist, who may recommend a *laparoscopy*. A minor procedure, it enables the uterus, tubes and ovaries to be viewed through a telescope-like instrument with a lighting system incorporated into it. You will either be booked in as a day patient or stay for one or two nights. On the day you will be given an anaesthetic, usually general. A small incision (1–2 cms/½–¾ inch) is made just below the navel, and the abdomen is then inflated with carbon dioxide gas. This moves the intestines out of the way and gives a clearer view of the pelvis. When there is sufficient gas inside, the laparoscope is put through the same hole. The pelvis is looked at thoroughly, and the ovaries, tubes and uterus examined for disease. After the operation you may feel some discomfort for a day or so in the abdomen or shoulder tip (referred pain from the stretched diaphragm).

Pain in the lower abdomen is frequently due to bowel trouble, but this can't really be seen with a laparoscopy. If your pelvis looks normal then this is most likely to be the problem.

LAPAROSCOPY

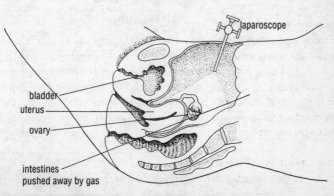

laparoscope

bladder
uterus
ovary

intestines
pushed away by gas

HEAVY PERIODS (*Menorrhagia*)

It's very difficult to gauge if you've got heavy periods – you only have yourself to compare with, it's not easy to measure how much blood you're losing, and what's normal for you may well be very heavy for someone else.

Most women bleed every twenty-one to thirty-five days for anywhere between two to seven days. The average blood loss is about 35 ml/ 1¼ fl oz per period. Anything over 80 ml/3 fl oz is said to be heavy, but this isn't easy to judge.

Some doctors use a menstrual blood loss chart (see diagram) to help you and them see how heavy your periods are. It can also assess the effect of any treatment, to see if things are getting worse or better, or if your periods are just the same. After initial instruction from your doctor you can monitor your blood loss each month and keep a record for her to see. The charts can be used whether you're using pads or tampons or both. Many women find their periods getting a little heavier in their thirties and forties, especially if they have had a baby or two, so this is perfectly normal.

For some women, on the other hand, it is quite normal to bleed only once or twice a year (often it will run in the family). As this means they may produce only a few eggs a year, they may need help if they're trying for a baby.

About one in five women are worried about their loss and seek medical help.

MENSTRUAL BLOOD LOSS CHART

Towel		1	2	3	4	5	6	7	8
	▭	II	I	I	IIII	II	I		
	▭		III	IIII	III	I			
	▭	I							
	clots		50pxI	IpxI					
	flooding								
Tampon	▭	I	I	I	I	I			
	▭		II	I	III	II			
	▭		II	II					
	clots								
	flooding		x2						

What causes heavy periods?

Hormones For most women under forty there will be no physical reason. The cause is then hormonal and called *dysfunctional uterine bleeding*. Some women will fail to ovulate properly, go for long periods without a period and then have a very heavy one. More commonly, however, the periods are regular and happen in normal ovulatory cycles. In fact, hormone levels are also usually perfectly normal.

Prostaglandins – the tissue hormones that have been blamed for painful periods – also play a part in heavy periods. Women with heavy periods have increased levels of prostaglandins, although no one has yet discovered why.

Fibroids/Polyps Occasionally there is a problem such as fibroids (page 56) or a polyp (page 57) causing the bleeding; fibroids come from the uterine muscle and polyps from the lining of the uterus (endometrial polyp) or cervix. These are benign (non-cancerous) growths. They make you bleed more as they make the surface area of the endometrium (uterine lining) larger.

Endometriosis/pelvic inflammatory disease Heavy bleeding also goes with the chronic pain of pelvic inflammatory disease (PID, page 59) and endometriosis (page 57).

In extremely rare cases, the endometrium will have a small cancer or pre-cancerous changes.

Treatment for menorrhagia

If you are at all worried about your loss go and see your doctor with details of your periods (see opposite). She will want to know if you are anaemic – feeling tired and washed out. If there is any doubt, she will take a blood sample to be checked for its haemoglobin level and maybe a test of your iron stores.

Your doctor may first want to try you on some simple drugs before sending you to a gynaecologist. She may try to reduce your prostaglandin levels with anti-prostaglandin tablets (Ponstan). You will need to begin taking the tablets the day before each period starts (not always easy to pinpoint with accuracy) and continue them for as long as your periods are heavy.

Progestogen drugs (Primulot, Provera) act like the hormone progesterone and seem to help control the bleeding even if you're not short of progesterone. They are particularly helpful if you're not ovulating properly and your cycles are very irregular. The tablets are usually taken for two to three weeks out of each four-week cycle.

DILATATION AND CURETTAGE (D&C) If the bleeding carries on being heavy a D & C is often recommended to check for any physical cause. This is a minor operation and takes about five minutes. Under a general anaesthetic, first the vulva and vagina are cleaned, and then the pelvis examined (easier to do when you're asleep and completely relaxed). The shape, size and position of the uterus are felt, as well as the ovaries on either side. The cervix is then opened a little (dilated) with graduated metal rods and a long, thin metal instrument with a spoonlike end (curette) inserted to scrape the lining of the uterus. The tissue is brought down to the cervix into the vagina and then sent to the laboratory for testing.

DILATATION AND CURETTAGE

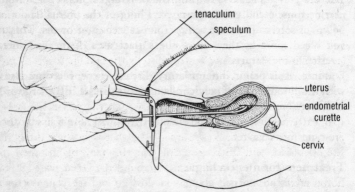

HYSTEROSCOPY This involves passing a small telescope through the cervix and is useful for spotting polyps or fibroids in the uterus. It's sometimes done at the same time as a D & C depending on the hospital.

If the D & C is normal, together with the result from the laboratory, and your periods are still bad, other therapies are available. A D & C isn't designed to improve things, but it quite often does, perhaps in a psychological way – conversely, stress can make periods worse.

THE PILL This can be useful for the younger woman (page 64) and can help to reduce the blood loss.

HORMONE REPLACEMENT THERAPY Similarly, hormone replacement therapy (HRT) may benefit the older woman nearing the menopause.

OTHER DRUGS Danazol (Danol) and buserilin (Suprefact) are sometimes prescribed. Both interfere with ovarian activity and can abolish periods altogether. Because they have other side-effects, they are not suitable for long-term use.

What's new
About one in five women ends up having a hysterectomy (see below) – a good proportion of these for heavy periods without a physical cause. Recently, pathologists looked at all the hysterectomy specimens in one study and found half of them were entirely normal.

The problem with heavy periods seems to be confined to the inner surface layer alone, the endometrium. Why can't just that bit of the uterus be removed? It could potentially save thousands of major operations.

ENDOMETRIAL RESECTION A new way of helping women with heavy periods has recently been developed along these lines, the aim being to destroy the endometrium alone. This whole concept is still under trial, but first results look very promising. A good proportion of women don't see any periods again, some have lighter, more bearable periods.

In this technique the endometrium is either burnt out with a very hot wire loop or vaporised away with a laser. Then, when the next menstrual cycle starts and oestrogen tells the endometrium to grow in readiness for a fertilised egg, there is nothing to grow. Newer, perhaps technically easier, techniques are being developed using microwaves.

An endometrial resection is done through the cervix like a D & C (page 50) and takes about thirty to forty minutes. Fluid has to circulate around the uterus to help the surgeon see what he or she is doing during the operation, and initial concern that this may be absorbed in any significant quantity now seems unfounded. Great care is taken, however, to check this.

If the burn is done too deeply, it will burn a hole right through the uterus, which usually means a hysterectomy is done there and then (this doesn't happen often). However, you should be prepared for a hysterectomy in the event that you are the one case that is difficult.

The endometrial resection means only a short hospital stay, and some units are doing it as day case surgery.

Afterwards, most women have one more heavy period and then that's it. Some go on with regular periods which are very much lighter, some stay the same. It does not work as a contraceptive until you've had at least a year without a period.

HYSTERECTOMY

Despite the new advances, *hysterectomy* still plays an important part in dealing with women's problems – over 1000 women each week have hysterectomies in this country, many more in America. It is a very effective operation if done for the right reasons at the right time. However, some women have rightly questioned the number of hysterectomies performed, and whether they have all been necessary. In particular, women in their forties have reported being pressurised into having one when there was nothing seriously wrong. It is important, therefore, if your consultant suggests you have a hysterectomy, to run through a checklist of questions.

– Why do I need one?
– Is there any alternative?
– Does it have to be done now?
– Will it be through the abdomen or vagina?
– Will you remove the ovaries as well?
– Is there any risk of particular complications?
– How long is the hospital stay?
– When will I be recovered – fit to drive, go back to work?
– What's the waiting list like?

In a busy hospital clinic it can be very upsetting to be told you need a major operation, your name has been put on the waiting list and that's that. You may find yourself outside in the corridor bewildered and confused, and later angry or afraid or both if you haven't understood why the operation is necessary. When you go to see the consultant take a friend or your partner with you for support, and take your list of questions. Ask the most important ones first, and write down the answers. Many departments have specially produced leaflets explaining the operation and what to expect. Ask if one's available.

Be sure in your own mind that this is the right thing for you, that you're in control of the situation and that all the other options have been explored. Women have found it very difficult to come to terms with themselves after a hysterectomy when they haven't had a clear idea of why it was being done, or if the decision was made in haste, without looking at the alternatives. It is a major operation that shouldn't be embarked on lightly for any woman. A woman loses her fertility when the uterus is removed, and for some this itself can be a difficult psychological event. For women who have interests outside the home and children already, this aspect isn't usually a problem; for others it can be traumatic, especially if they haven't clearly understood what a hysterectomy involves. If you're not happy with the consultant's diagnosis talk it over with your GP. She may well be able to reassure you or suggest a second opinion.

When is a hysterectomy necessary?

Dysfunctional uterine bleeding When drug treatment fails to stop heavy periods and when the new endometrial resection operation is not suitable or available (page 51).

Fibroids These are muscle bundles which grow in the uterus and can make periods heavy (page 56).

Endometriosis Growths of endometrium (uterine lining) inside the uterine muscle, on the ovaries and tubes and elsewhere can cause pelvic pain and painful heavy periods (page 57).

Chronic pelvic inflammatory disease This can also make the pelvis sore and the periods heavy (page 59).

Cancer When there is cancer of the cervix, endometrium (lining of the uterus) and ovary. Each requires a specific type of hysterectomy.

Prolapse of the uterus Usually causes a lump in the vagina, which can be uncomfortable, and is not improved by pelvic floor exercises (see page 177).

What's involved

A hysterectomy is the removal of the uterus. It is called a *total hysterectomy* if the cervix is removed, and a *sub-total* or *partial hysterectomy* if the cervix stays behind as a stump. Most hysterectomies are total ones. Leaving a bit of cervix behind means you still need regular cervical smears. If the ovaries and tubes are also removed it's called a *hysterectomy and a bilateral* (both sides) *salpingo-oophorectomy*. If it is necessary to take more of the surrounding tissue, including the glands, as in cancer of the cervix or endometrium, the operation is called a *Wertheim's* or *radical hysterectomy*.

HYSTERECTOMY

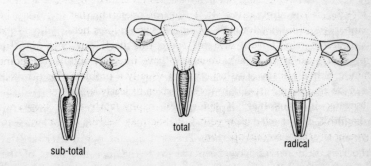

sub-total   total   radical

There are two main ways of doing a hysterectomy: through the abdomen or through the vagina. Usually the vaginal way is reserved for women with prolapse – a weakness in the supports of the uterus causing a swelling in the vagina (page 177)

ABDOMINAL HYSTERECTOMY This is done through a bikini incision straight across the abdomen. The uterus and cervix are removed, and sometimes the ovaries and tubes, too. Ask your surgeon, you may need hormone replacement therapy if the ovaries are removed.

VAGINAL HYSTERECTOMY This is done through a cut in the vagina. The uterus and cervix are removed and the walls of the vagina strengthened and tightened.

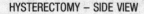

HYSTERECTOMY – SIDE VIEW

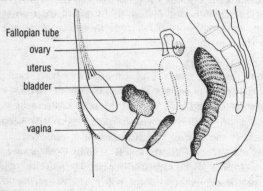

Fallopian tube
ovary
uterus
bladder

vagina

Afterwards

You may wake up with a drip in your arm and a catheter tube draining the bladder. Within a couple of days you will be up and about and can expect to go home after about a week.

Expect to be tired, very tired, when you get home. Just because you're fit to go home doesn't mean you can take on looking after the family where you left off. This is a good reason for staying in hospital longer, but most women are very ready to go home after a week.

You will have bleeding for about seven to ten days as the vaginal stitches heal. The loss shouldn't be heavy and needs to be reported if it is. The skin, whether stapled together, stitched on the inside or outside, will be healed after a week. The internal stitches take longer as the muscle layer knits together. The skin may be numb afterwards as the tiny skin nerves have been cut with the incision; most of the sensation comes back in time. You may have lost some blood at the operation and need to take iron tablets when you go home.

Take things easy for about a month: rest as soon as you feel tired. Leave driving until your wound is comfortable and not pulling, usually after about a month. Avoid any heavy lifting, including kettles and saucepans, in this first month.

Sex, if it was good before, is very likely to be good (or better) again after the operation – if you've been suffering pain or heavy periods you can at last enjoy sex again, with no fear of pregnancy either. Wait a month before you try it, though. Take it very gently the first few times and use a lubricating cream (KY jelly) to make it easier.

The vagina, whether you have an abdominal or vaginal hysterectomy, will be sewn up securely. This is well healed after four weeks. The clitoris and surrounding labia are untouched in a hysterectomy. Those women who could feel the deep thrusts of their partner's penis touching the cervix will not do so after a hysterectomy as the vagina is sewn over at the top.

The long term

A hysterectomy is a major operation so don't be surprised if you're still exhausted six months after the operation – if you can, indulge yourself, get up later, have an afternoon nap, and don't feel guilty about needing more rest.

You won't get periods any more, but if your ovaries are left behind you may still experience monthly mood swings or even premenstrual syndrome. The menopause will be a few years earlier, so your risk of coronary heart disease goes up after the operation until other women catch you up at fifty. Don't forget to do your pelvic floor exercises (page 150). It's just as important to keep the vagina toned up and the bladder and rectum nicely supported.

In one study of women following hysterectomy, 90 per cent were satisfied with the end result, so for many it's the right operation.

> *I had problems for eight or nine years. My periods just got worse and worse. I would flood with no warning, I couldn't go anywhere and it was so embarrassing as I work in an office with men.*
>
> *I saw doctors on and off for years and specialists, but I really didn't like to keep bothering them. I had several D&Cs and they tried various pills but nothing worked. Finally, in January this year, I just couldn't stand it any longer and saw the consultant*

who told me that the only option was a hysterectomy. I didn't mind, I was quite happy to go through with it. I didn't want any more children – my husband had in fact had a vasectomy.

I went into hospital in April. I was very relaxed, I had a total hysterectomy which meant an incision in my tummy. My stomach was very sore for about two weeks and then it just got stronger and stronger. I'm back at work now after three months off. I feel fine. I would certainly recommend it. People told me to expect emotional problems, but I have had none at all.

Women's Health, 52 Featherstone Street, London EC1Y 8RT. Tel: 071–251 6580. Send s.a.e. for publication list.

UTERINE DISORDERS

FIBROIDS (*Myoma*)

These are bundles of muscle that grow in the muscle wall of the uterus (*myometrium*). About one in five women will have one or more fibroids by the time she's forty, so they're quite common. A fibroid starts off as a tiny, pea-sized lump and can grow to the size of a grapefruit or even larger. They are not cancerous and many women don't even know they have them. It is the oestrogen in our bodies that makes fibroids grow, but the combined Pill doesn't have any effect as its oestrogen is balanced by a progestogen. After the menopause fibroids shrink.

If the fibroid is near the inner lining of the uterus (*endometrium*) it will stretch it and make a larger surface area from which to bleed each month. Fibroids can grow sufficiently big to make your abdomen stick out, just as a pregnancy would. Fibroids can cause pressure effects on

FIBROIDS

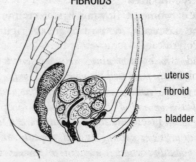

uterus
fibroid
bladder

the bladder, with incontinence and making it necessary to pass urine frequently; or on the pelvic veins, giving you varicose veins, piles or leg swelling. They can make you generally uncomfortable, with backache which is often worse with a period.

Fibroids can be associated with difficulty in conceiving, but it's not clear why; it is possible that pregnancy protects you from developing fibroids rather than the other way round. They're certainly more common in women who have never been pregnant.

Fibroids occasionally dissolve their centres and break down. This is sometimes very painful, especially when it happens in pregnancy.

DIAGNOSIS A careful bimanual pelvic examination will pick up moderately enlarged fibroids (approximately plum-sized). An ultrasound scan (page 112) can help to confirm they are there.

TREATMENT None, if the fibroids are small and not causing any problems. If you want to conceive and the fibroids are thought to be distorting the uterine cavity, a simple operation to remove them (*myomectomy*) may be suggested.

If you do not want to have any more children and there are period problems or pressure problems in the pelvic area, the sensible solution is probably a hysterectomy. Drugs to reduce oestrogen levels work while you take them, but these can't be used indefinitely because of the risk of osteoporosis and the fibroids grow back as soon as you stop.

POLYPS

Polyps are tube-like growths that can appear in the lining of the uterus (*endometrial polyps*) or cervix (*cervical polyps*). They are not cancerous, but can cause irregular bleeding between periods or after intercourse.

DIAGNOSIS Any unusual bleeding should be reported to your doctor. A polyp on the cervix may be visible during an examination; endometrial polyps are hidden away inside the uterus and are usually only found at a D & C (page 50). They sometimes occur if the hormone balance isn't right in the years coming up to the menopause.

TREATMENT Polyps can be removed under a local anaesthetic. They are twisted off and the bases sealed with an electric cautery needle. Endometrial polyps are removed by a D & C.

ENDOMETRIOSIS

This is a strange condition where the lining of the uterus (*endometrium*) is actually outside the uterus — it can appear as little spots on the ovaries, tubes, the supporting ligaments of the uterus, the bowel and the bladder and in the muscle layer of the uterus itself. The problem is the monthly bleed: these spots of endometrium behave just like the endometrium lining the uterus, growing under hormone control and bleeding every month at period time. The body tissues react to this irritating blood by getting inflamed and forming scar tissue. Periods can be very painful for some women with this problem. The inflammation can give constant discomfort, not just at period time, and make intercourse very sore. When you're examined the doctor may be able to feel nodules of inflammation and it all may be generally tender inside at the top of the vagina.

About 1–2 per cent of women have endometriosis, many without knowing it. For some reason it's more common in women in the higher socioeconomic groups and in women who've only had one or two children or none at all. Pregnancy may therefore protect you from endometriosis. It appears mainly between the ages of thirty and forty-five.

There are many theories about why endometriosis occurs. One is that when certain women menstruate, the blood not only comes out of the vagina but also goes up the Fallopian tubes and spills into the peritoneal cavity in the abdomen. This, in fact, happens in many women but they don't all have endometriosis. It also doesn't explain the very rare times when endometriotic spots appear in the lungs. Another explanation is that tiny bits of endometrium pass into the blood stream or lymphatic system and are sent to various parts of the pelvis. Possibly the problem stems from hormonal imbalance.

ENDOMETRIOSIS – COMMON SITES

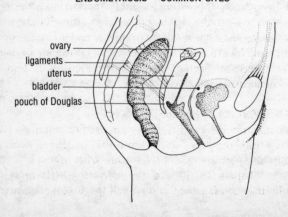

ovary
ligaments
uterus
bladder
pouch of Douglas

Endometriosis is associated with difficulties in conceiving.

DIAGNOSIS A laparoscopy (page 47) makes diagnosis very easy.

TREATMENT If the endometriosis is mild, drugs can be given to simulate pregnancy – the contraceptive Pill and progestogens (Duphaston) – or the menopause – danazol (Danol) and the nasal spray buserilin (Suprefact). Either way your hormones are on a plateau which prevents the monthly stimulation of the uterus lining. The aim is to stop your periods and if the treatment is not doing this it must be altered.

You should carry on with treatment for at least six months to allow the areas of endometriosis to shrink and disappear. There is a chance though that the endometriosis will need further treatment sometime in the future.

What's new

The laser can vaporise spots of endometriosis and will possibly give results as good as drug treatment. This is done at the same time as a laparoscopy. It can also cut away any scar tissue that has formed. This requires considerable skill and is only available in some hospitals. Research is underway to see if laser treatment can improve fertility rates and pain levels better than conventional drug treatment.

Severe disease The tubes and ovaries can be badly damaged by endometriosis, preventing ovulation and the normal wafting of the egg down the tube. At this stage, if you still want children the options become limited. Drug treatment may help to start with, followed by an operation to try to improve the position of the pelvic organs.

If you do not want any more children and drug treatment hasn't worked a hysterectomy (page 51) may be suggested. However, there is some controversy over the effectiveness of a hysterectomy in treating endometriosis. If only the uterus is removed, the ovaries will still produce oestrogen, possibly resulting in further endometriosis growths. Some consultants like to take the ovaries at the same time so that there are no more hormone swings each month. This will lead to an immediate menopause, and all the changes that go with it.

PELVIC INFLAMMATORY DISEASE (PID)

Pelvic inflammatory disease (PID) is a term used to describe a range of infections affecting the pelvic area. Acute PID is defined as an illness with a high temperature and pelvic pain with signs of a genital infection (see Chapter Three). As the infection travels upwards the inflammation may be diagnosed as cervicitis (page 31), endometritis in the uterus (page 57), or an infection in the tubes or in the ovaries.

Chronic PID can be the result of several infections in the past. Chlamydia and gonorrhoea are often the bacteria that do the initial damage, paving the way for less harmful infections to enter and cause further trouble. It seems the first infection makes the Fallopian tubes and ovaries more vulnerable to any sort of infection.

The inflammation grumbles on leaving you with heavy, painful periods: abnormal vaginal discharge; backache; painful intercourse, possibly with bleeding; problems with urinating; a swollen abdomen; and a general feeling of being unwell.

DIAGNOSIS A vaginal examination will show a discharge coming from the cervix if an infection is present, the ovaries and uterus may not move in the normal way, and everything may be very tender. A swab taken from the cervix sometimes shows infection but not always.

A laparoscopy (page 47) is often done to find out the cause of the pain; the symptoms can be very like those of endometriosis (page 57).

TREATMENT Antibiotics are prescribed, and can be effective if the infection is treated early enough. If the problems continue, however, and if you want children, the best results come with surgery. Very fine adhesions can be divided with laser or diathermy through the laparoscope, but any more than this needs microsurgery.

If you don't get pregnant after this procedure then the next bet is to try for an IVF pregnancy (test tube baby, page 144). This bypasses your tubes altogether, but unfortunately is not widely available on the NHS.

If you do not want any more children and the pain and difficult periods are making your life a misery, a hysterectomy (page 51) may be the best solution. If you're unhappy with this idea and don't feel ready for such radical surgery, alternative pain-relieving treatments such as acupuncture (page 23) may help and are worth considering.

CANCER OF THE CERVIX

This is the commonest cancer of the genitals. Women in their fifties are most likely to be diagnosed as suffering from cervical cancer. Women who have had children and those who've had many sexual partners are more at risk. So are smokers. For some reason, Jewish women rarely get cervical cancer (perhaps related to their husbands being circumcised, or simply that they have fewer sexual partners, no one is really sure).

The symptoms can vary from none at all, to abnormal bleeding after intercourse or between periods, brown smelly vaginal discharge and bladder upset.

DIAGNOSIS A routine cervical smear; a colposcopy (page 32) will show the abnormal area clearly, and taking a tissue sample (biopsy) will confirm if there is cancer of the cervix.

TREATMENT Usually radiotherapy, but if the cancer is found at an early stage, surgery is considered. The uterus, cervix and top part of the vagina are removed but the ovaries can be spared. This is called a *Wertheim's hysterectomy*, and extra glandular tissue is removed to assess the spread of the disease. Survival rates for surgery and radiotherapy are very similar for very early cancers.

OUTLOOK Very good (90 per cent survive for at least five years) if the cancer is discovered early. Cervical smear screening has helped to pick up early cases and has improved survival rates.

CANCER OF THE UTERUS (ENDOMETRIAL CANCER)

Cancer of the uterus mainly affects women in their fifties and over, usually causing bleeding after the menopause. The cancer develops in the lining of the uterus. It's more common in overweight women and those with high blood pressure or diabetes. Women who've never had children are also more at risk. It is related to oestrogen levels, and originally HRT (page 171), which gave oestrogen alone, caused an increase in endometrial cancer.

DIAGNOSIS The most common symptom is bleeding after the menopause. In women still menstruating irregular bleeding between periods or a watery discharge can be the only indications. A D & C (page 50) is necessary to confirm the diagnosis, and a tissue sample sent to the laboratory for testing.

TREATMENT Standard treatment is an extended, or radical, hysterectomy (page 53). Extra radiotherapy may be necessary if the cancer shows any signs of spreading. Progestogens (Provera) are useful to dampen down the tumour in advanced cases.

OUTLOOK Good, because the bleeding is an excellent early warning sign. If the cancer is limited to the uterus itself, as it usually is, the survival rate to five years is above 75 per cent.

OVARIAN CYSTS

Ovarian cysts are quite common and are usually a by-product of the ovulation process. Symptoms can often be nothing at all, or discomfort and/or swelling in the lower abdomen, pain during intercourse, and irregularities in the menstrual cycle.

DIAGNOSIS Cysts are usually discovered during a pelvic examination.

TREATMENT Ultrasound scanning is very helpful in checking on the size of a cyst. Sometimes if the cyst is small it will disappear of its own accord, but if it continues to grow or causes trouble (twisting or bleeding) it can either be drained (usually through a laparoscope) or removed surgically. It doesn't mean you lose your ovary as once the cyst is removed the ovary can usually be restored.

OVARIAN CANCER

This is much more common in the Western industrialised countries. It is generally found in women in their fifties and sixties. Pregnancy (the earlier the better) protects you and so does the Pill. If your mother or sister has had cancer of the ovary then you have a greater risk of getting it. If you've had cancer of the breast, bowel or uterus your risk is also increased. Talcum powder has been blamed for causing ovarian cancer; it's best not used on sanitary towels or for dusting between your legs.

DIAGNOSIS Feeling bloated and discomfort in your abdomen may be your only symptoms, as a tumour of the ovary can grow quite large without causing any trouble at all. Your doctor may be able to feel an enlarged ovary during a pelvic examination. Tests may include an ultrasound scan and blood tests.

TREATMENT Usually involves surgery to remove the growth, and taking the uterus and the other ovary at the same time. If the growth has spread inside, chemotherapy is given after recovery from the operation.

OUTLOOK Very good if picked up early. Often, though, the cancer will have spread in the abdomen and then advice about the future must be guarded.

What's new

Because ovarian cancer is discovered late, screening tests for an early diagnosis would be ideal. So far, scanning ovaries, blood tests for cancer proteins, and regular examinations have been on trial. None has yet provided the complete answer, which means that we must rely on a pelvic examination at the time of taking a smear.

If you're at risk (someone in the family has already had the disease) ask your doctor about having your ovaries screened. If you do not want any more children it may be worth considering having your ovaries removed (you would need hormone replacement therapy afterwards).

—3—

SEX AND THE CONSEQUENCES

Today's women have a freedom to enjoy life and their sexuality in a way unheard of earlier this century. The coming of the Pill in the 1960s coincided with more liberal thinking in general and contributed to a greater openness about sex and sex education.

Despite this there are casualties – girls with unwanted pregnancies, or with sexually transmitted diseases. Now, too, there is the looming epidemic of AIDS. The best you can do is practise safe sex with good contraception in a loving stable relationship and no risk taking.

CONTRACEPTION

From our teens to our fifties, contraception helps us to be in control of our bodies and our sexuality. It means we can choose whether we want to have children and when we want them. Many of us have jobs we enjoy, some with a career structure, some to provide much needed extra money. We need to have control over our lives, to enjoy sex without worrying about unwanted pregnancies or sexually transmitted diseases. Mistakes will still happen, but we can choose a method of contraception that minimises the risks, depending on our lifestyle, age and health.

Why bother with contraception?

If a young couple are having regular sexual intercourse and using no contraception for a year the chances of getting pregnant are in the region of 80–90 per cent.

The reproductive system is designed to seize every opportunity of achieving a pregnancy. Many women feel greatest desire at the most fertile time of the month, usually from about the eleventh to the seventeenth day in a twenty-eight-day cycle, when the cervical mucus is more fluid and welcoming to sperm. The cervix itself is actually higher up in the vagina at ovulation and is softer and slightly open. This is good news for the swimming sperm deposited at the top of the vagina.

And there are enough of them. With each ejaculation of say 4 ml (about a dessertspoon) there can be as many as 400 million sperm. All this to fertilise one egg! The sperm can survive for as long as four or five days in the right mucus. The egg only lives for twenty-four hours.

In a twenty-eight-day menstrual cycle with ovulation occurring on day fourteen, the fertile phase can last from day nine to day fifteen. Unfortunately, this time can be very variable, being shorter or much longer.

The ideal method of contraception would guarantee no chance of pregnancy. It wouldn't interfere with intercourse. It would be quite safe, with no side-effects, and you could stop it to get pregnant when you wanted. Unfortunately, nothing quite fits the bill yet, but current research into contraception is investigating lots of interesting ideas. The options available at present suit a variety of women with different lifestyles and requirements.

THE COMBINED PILL
WHAT IT IS The combined Pill contains two hormones, man-made oestrogen and progestogen compounds. Progestogens are artificial hormones which act like progesterone (pure progesterone can't be taken by mouth). Newer versions of progestogens (desogestrel, gestodene) have less effect on fat metabolism and may reduce the risks of serious heart and circulatory problems.

Phased pills contain oestrogen and progestogen hormones in different amounts throughout the cycle. The idea is to mimic the normal menstrual cycle, keeping the hormone levels as low as possible. They also help with difficult breakthrough bleeding. Because of the varying hormone levels throughout the month, pill-taking errors are more common, especially when there's been a missed pill. Some women find they have premenstrual symptoms with this Pill.

HOW IT WORKS The combined Pill stops ovulation, makes the cervical mucus inhospitable to sperm and possibly affects the wafting movement in the Fallopian tube that encourages the egg and sperm to meet.

HOW IT IS TAKEN By mouth. Most types of Pill work round a four-week cycle, taking the Pill for twenty-one days with a seven-day break for withdrawal bleeding, which is usually like a light period.

You can start the Pill on the first day of menstruation and be protected straight away. Your next period will come early, and the ones after that will be on a twenty-eight-day cycle. It is a good idea to have a regular time for taking the Pill, so it becomes part of your routine and easy to remember. It is not essential to take the Pill at exactly the same time every day – within four to six hours is sensible.

If you want to avoid a withdrawal bleed in any particular month, you can take two packets continuously without a break (but not with the phased Pill).

There is quite often spotting (breathrough bleeding) between periods at the beginning and some women experience nausea and breast tenderness. These usually settle down with time, but if they don't the Pill needs to be changed. Don't stop taking the tablets if you have breakthrough bleeding. Never stop the Pill without using another form of contraception.

MISSED PILLS Because the Pill works by delivering a small daily amount of hormone it is important not to miss one. If you forget and remember within twelve hours of when the Pill should have been taken take the tablet at once and the next one at the time it is normally due. Assume everything is okay. If it's longer than twelve hours, take the following precautions. If you forget a pill or have an attack of diarrhoea and vomiting in the first fourteen days of the pill-taking cycle, take the missed Pill (or two if you've missed several), and carry on taking the pills. Use extra precautions (sheath and spermicide) for the next seven days. If pills are missed in the last seven days, forget the seven-day break and start a new packet of pills after the old one is finished. Do this regardless of any bleeding. You should always check this with your doctor.

FAILURE RATE Less than 1 per cent if taken correctly: every day without fail, apart from the pill-free period, and taking precautions (see above) if a Pill is missed. It is the most reliable, easily reversible method of contraception.

IS IT FOR YOU? If you have ever had any blood clots or blood disorders, certain liver conditions, breast cancer or heart disesase then it's not for you. If you're a diabetic, the pill can upset your insulin balance; the progestogen-only Pill may be better if you want oral contraception. Particular care must be taken if you're fat, smoke, have ever had raised blood pressure or suffer with migraine. It is fine for women who have had a colposcopy and treatment for *cervical intrepithelial neoplasia* (CIN, page 32) to carry on taking the Pill.

If you smoke, the Pill is not suitable over the age of thirty-five. Smoking increases the risk of having a stroke or heart attack. You should give up if you are under thirty-five and considering the Pill.

Some women naturally have irregular periods. The Pill may not be the best for them as they may find there is a delay in the return of their periods, which can be upsetting if they then want a baby.

Taking the Pill beyond the age of forty does carry a higher risk of heart attack and stroke (made worse by smoking). The risk of blood clots goes up, too. This must be fully discussed with your doctor. A low-dose Pill (Mercilon) may be suitable.

WHERE TO GET THE PILL It is available from your doctor or a family planning clinic. To find your nearest clinic, ask your GP or look it up in the phone book under 'Family Planning'. You should phone up to check whether you need to make an appointment, although some clinics still operate on a walk-in basis.

WHEN THE PILL IS PRESCRIBED It is a very good idea to have a general examination to check your blood pressure, body weight and have your breasts examined. It is not always necessary to have an internal examination, but if you are due to have a smear then it's best done then.

ADVANTAGES If you suffer from heavy, painful periods, the Pill can improve affairs to give a lightish, shorter bleed. Mood swings and premenstrual tension quite often improve as well. It seems to protect against cancers of the ovary and endometrium. There is also a reduced risk of pelvic inflammatory disease (the thicker mucus in the cervix stops both sperm and germs). Ovarian cysts, benign breast lumps, rheumatoid arthritis and thyroid trouble are all less common if you're on the Pill. It can improve your skin if you have acne.

The combined Pill is easy to use, extremely reliable and doesn't interfere with love-making.

DISADVANTAGES AND SIDE-EFFECTS You may feel nauseous at first, although this usually clears up after a few weeks. Taking the Pill at night may help. You may put on weight due to water retention; your ankles may swell and some women find their contact lenses become irritating. Some women experience mood changes and depression, which in turn could affect your desire for sex. You may also find your vagina is drier and sex uncomfortable; a lubricant (KY jelly) should improve this.

More serious side-effects include developing blood clots and high blood pressure, leading to a heart attack or a stroke; the risk is increased if you smoke or are overweight. Women who have a close family member with diabetes or who have had a large baby (greater than 4.5 kg/10 lb) may be diabetics-in-waiting and the Pill could act as a trigger. If you're likely to suffer with gall-stones sometime in your life, the Pill can make it happen earlier. Some women develop severe headaches and migraine whilst taking the Pill. It is usually best to stop if this is the case. If you develop any liver problems the Pill must be stopped. There is some evidence that the Pill may alter the immune system in some women, making them more prone to certain viral illnesses.

The phased Pill may cause ovarian cysts (page 61). They usually disappear if the phased Pill is stopped.

There has been much controversy about breast cancer, but the latest medical opinion is that the Pill doesn't increase the risk. Some studies have suggested that prolonged use under the age of twenty-five or before having a baby may increase the chances of early breast cancer, but this hasn't been confirmed.

The Pill does not protect you from sexually transmitted diseases, so condoms are essential if you're in any doubt about your partner's past sexual life or if you have many partners.

THE PROGESTOGEN-ONLY PILL (POP or Mini-pill)

WHAT IT IS This pill contains only progestogen. It's taken every day – at the same time each day – without a break.

HOW IT WORKS The Mini-pill makes the cervical mucus thicker and more difficult for the sperms to penetrate. It also changes the lining of the uterus so that the fertilised egg will not implant itself. The normal wafting movement in the tubes is probably disturbed, too.

HOW TO TAKE THE MINI-PILL If you normally have intercourse when you go to bed at night, the best time to take the Mini-pill is early evening (the effect on the cervical mucus wears off quite soon), *not* just before bedtime (this means relying on the pill taken the night before). To work effectively it must be taken at the same time every day within an hour, preferably early evening, but if this is not convenient or your love-making times vary choose a regular time that suits you.

MISSED PILLS Forgetting a pill, even if it's only three hours late, means it will not work. The missed Pill should be taken as soon as possible, and a barrier method of contraception used for the next forty-eight hours. Continue to take the pills as normal. If you miss two or more pills visit your doctor for emergency contraception.

FAILURE RATE If taken properly the failure rate is about 2–3 per cent. This decreases in older women (1% over thirty-five, 0.3% over forty).

IS IT FOR YOU? As the amount of hormone taken is much less, the progestogen-only pill can be taken by more women than the combined

Pill. It is suitable for women over thirty-five who smoke, diabetics and women who have had blood clots or high blood pressure. Women who want a hormonal method and are breastfeeding can also take it. It is a very good method for the reliable pill-taker who only wants to take the smallest amount of extra hormone.

The Mini-pill is probably not suitable for women who have breast cancer or any other cancers of the reproductive system. If you have had any problems with pelvic inflammatory disease or had an ectopic pregnancy, it is also not recommended. If you have any problems with your liver, the Mini-pill will not be considered.

ADVANTAGES The Mini-pill can improve your periods if they're painful, and help some women with premenstrual tension. As with the combined Pill, the hostile cervical mucus gives some protection against pelvic inflammatory disease, as it keeps the germs out as well. It is a very good method if you are well organised and have a good memory. If you're forgetful and disorganised, another contraceptive method would be better. It has fewer of the serious complications of the combined Pill and can be used up to the menopause.

DISADVANTAGES AND SIDE-EFFECTS Periods may become irregular, and some even missed altogether; bleeding in the middle of the cycle is not unusual. In fact, probably the more irregular the cycle the more effective the contraception. There's a slightly higher risk of an ectopic pregnancy (page 118) because of the changes in the tube function. This also applies to cysts in the ovary (page 61), perhaps because of a minor change in ovulation. This method only gives slight protection against some sexually transmitted diseases, but none against HIV.

REVERSIBILITY Often fertility returns in the next cycle. Ovulation may be delayed a little with the combined Pill. It certainly doesn't matter if you get pregnant straight away – ultrasound scanning can usually sort out any problems with dating the pregnancy.

INTRA-UTERINE DEVICE (IUD OR COIL)

WHAT IT IS The IUD is a small plastic device that sits in the uterus with a thread hanging down into the vagina. The plastic carries either copper or silver wire, or hormones.

HOW IT WORKS The IUD acts like a foreign body in the uterus, setting up a tissue reaction that prevents the fertilised egg from implanting and may also stop sperm getting to the egg in the first place. The steroid IUDs (containing progestogen) affect the cervical mucus, also making it inhospitable to sperm.

INTRA-UTERINE DEVICES

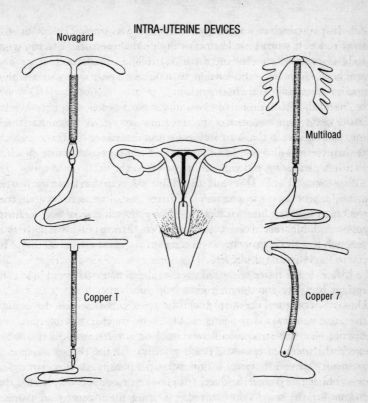

Novagard

Multiload

Copper T

Copper 7

FAILURE RATE 1.5–3 per cent.

IS IT FOR YOU? Not if you have irregular bleeding that hasn't been sorted out, or have had a serious pelvic infection or an ectopic pregnancy at any time. If you've had your tubes operated on in the past or have any sign of an infection this method of contraception is not recommended. Heavy periods, endometriosis and fibroids are all good reason for not having an IUD. Care is needed if you have a heart murmur or are on steroid type drugs.

If your lifestyle makes you liable to an increased chance of pelvic infection – many partners, not much idea of their past sexual encounters – the IUD isn't suitable for you. Because there is an increased risk of infection if you have an IUD, it's not recommended for those who have never been pregnant.

WHERE TO GET AN IUD The IUD has to be fitted by an experienced family planning doctor. She will ask about your personal history: period details, past pregnancies, any gynaecological problems. The doctor will want to know when your last period was – the easiest time to insert an IUD is towards the end of a period; this also ensures you are not pregnant. A pelvic examination is done first (page 33) and a smear taken if necessary. If there is any hint of pelvic infection the IUD won't be inserted. You will usually stay in the same position (lying on your back, knees bent and wide apart) for the insertion. A speculum is put into the vagina, in the same way as for a smear, to see the cervix, which is then cleaned and steadied by a grasping forceps – this may pinch a little. A measuring rod is gently passed into the uterus to measure the inside cavity. The IUD is then passed into the uterus in a narrow plastic straw; as soon as it's in position it springs into place to fit securely and the plastic straw is withdrawn. This procedure can be a little uncomfortable. Each coil has one or two threads which hang down through the cervix into the top of the vagina. These are cut so that 2 to 3 cm (¾–1¼ inch) can be felt.

You can feel quite faint and even nauseous afterwards, so you may want a friend to come with you to help you home. It's best to take it slowly afterwards. There may well be some bleeding and discomfort over the next two days. This shouldn't be much, with bleeding no heavier than for a period; paracetamol or similar painkillers should settle the pain. Afterwards, practise feeling for the threads. Get in a position that you find easy for inserting tampons, such as squatting or with one leg on a chair, and feel with one or two fingers deep inside the vagina for the wiry nylon threads. (During intercourse your partner may notice them slightly, and if they are cut too short they may prick his penis.) Check the threads each month after a period to make sure the IUD is there and doing its job. If you feel something more solid than the threads it may mean the IUD has become dislodged and is coming down the cervix; see your doctor as soon as possible. This occurs in 10 per cent of women, usually with the first or second period after insertion.

Most IUD failures (pregnancies) happen within the first three months, usually because the IUD is not in the right place. To be on the safe side, use a spermicide as well in the first few months – the IUD will be checked by the doctor during this time in any case. If all is well, you wil probably be checked once a year.

Copper IUDs are the most commonly fitted and need to be replaced from time to time, usually every three to five years. Removing it is a quick and painless procedure, but alternative contraception must have been used for a week previously. Do not attempt to take it out yourself for whatever reason.

ADVANTAGES Once inserted the IUD is almost forgotten and it doesn't interfere with intercourse.

DISADVANTAGES AND SIDE-EFFECTS Heavier, more painful periods are a problem for one in ten women, troublesome enough to have the IUD removed. Quite often, however, this problem improves with time and it's worth waiting to see if things settle down over the first three months. Simple analgesics such as paracetamol or anti-prostaglandin drugs (Ponstan) may be helpful.

Some women find they have a heavier discharge with the IUD, and thrush can be a persistent problem.

The chance of pelvic infection is slightly increased, probably because bacteria find the route is made easier from the vagina to the Fallopian tubes. Infection is much more common, however, if there is more than one sexual partner. Any signs of infection in the tubes should be treated very seriously: it could cause permanent damage and affect your ability to conceive. If you have a temperature, low abdominal discomfort, especially with intercourse, and vaginal discharge, report this to your doctor straight away. Antibiotics will be prescribed and the IUD may be removed.

There is a slightly higher risk of ectopic pregnancy (see page 118) with the IUD. This is because the fertilised egg may implant in the Fallopian tube instead of the inhospitable endometrium.

The IUD gives no protection against any sexually transmitted infections, including HIV.

REVERSIBILITY All the major studies indicate that the IUD does not affect fertility once it is removed. However, there is always the slight concern of pelvic infection and its effect on the Fallopian tubes and therefore the ability to conceive. It is very important that the IUD is reserved for the right group of women, that it's carefully inserted and that regular checks are done.

ADVICE Because of these risks the IUD usually doesn't take first place in the contraceptive options. However, for those who are suitable and whom it suits, the IUD gives worry-free birth control.

What's new
A new coil has been developed which releases a progestogen hormone. This looks very promising, with a low failure rate and the likelihood it will improve heavy periods. Trials are not complete as yet.

THE DIAPHRAGM

Women have put various things into their vaginas for centuries – leaves, sponges, crocodile dung in ancient Egypt – to prevent sperm swimming up into the uterus. The diaphragm, or Dutch cap, became available in the 1920s and revolutionised women's lives as the first safe contraception; it dropped out of fashion with the arrival of the Pill and the IUD. However, more women today are returning to this method either because they are unhappy with the prospect of taking hormones indefinitely or of having an IUD.

WHAT IT IS The diaphragm is a soft rubber hemisphere with a sprung rim that sits at the top of the vagina. It is smeared with spermicide cream or jelly and inserted up to three hours before intercourse. After sex it must be left in for six hours. If there's a delay from when you put the diaphragm in to when you have sex, it's wise to use some more spermicide (pessary or easy to insert foams are available). You should do this anyway if you have intercourse again within the six-hour period.

HOW IT WORKS The diaphragm carries the spermicide cream to the cervical entrance and holds it there. It keeps the sperm away from the friendly cervical mucus and makes them stay in the vagina, where it is too acidic for them to survive for long. It prevents the sperm being sucked up into the cervix and uterus by orgasmic waves.

FAILURE RATE About 2–3 per cent but very much depends on the user.

IS IT FOR YOU? You must be quite relaxed about exploring your vulva and vagina and be absolutely vigilant about using the diaphragm every

INSERTING THE DIAPHRAGM

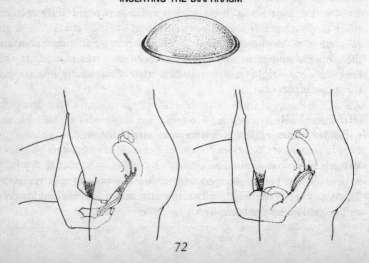

time. Women who have poor vaginal muscles or suffer from a prolapse (page 177) may not be suitable. If you're allergic to rubber then it's not for you (this is rare). It would be best for a virgin if her partner used a condom for the first few times of intercourse before being fitted for a diaphragm.

WHERE TO GET A DIAPHRAGM You can be fitted with a diaphragm at a family planning clinic or by your family doctor; clinics often have more time and facilities but general practices vary. Every woman is a different size, so the diaphragm needs to be fitted specially for you. You will be examined and various diaphragms tried to find the best fit. This doesn't hurt at all. You will be taught how to put it in and also how to apply the spermicide cream correctly. Usually you have a week to practise and then return to the clinic to see if you're doing it properly; use some other form of contraception in the meantime. Don't worry if it's difficult at first; it does get easier quite quickly.

The diaphragm must be kept clean and dry. Store it out of sunlight. Regularly check for holes and that it is not going out of shape. Unless you have any specific problems you should visit the clinic once a year for a check up, and make sure your diaphragm is changed every one or two years. Changes in your weight can mean your diaphragm won't fit properly any more – if you've put on or lost more than 3 kg (7 lb), had a baby or had a miscarriage or an abortion see your doctor as soon as possible to have your diaphragm checked.

ADVANTAGES Using the diaphragm is completely under your control and it is only used when it's needed. It protects the cervix from developing cancer. It helps reduce the risk of pelvic infection and probably HIV (the AIDS virus is thought to be destroyed by spermicides). It has none of the serious side-effects of the Pill or IUD.

DISADVANTAGES AND SIDE-EFFECTS Cystitis (page 28) is more common in diaphragm users, and some women develop an allergy to the spermicide. It does require a bit of forethought, and it's no good if it stays in the drawer.

THE CONDOM

In Roman times animal bladders were used as condoms to prevent sexually transmitted diseases. In the eighteenth century, sheep's bowel was used to protect against pregnancy. Advances in rubber technology in the middle of the last century made a dramatic difference to contraception. Worldwide, between thirty and forty million couples use the condom for contraception.

PUTTING ON A CONDOM

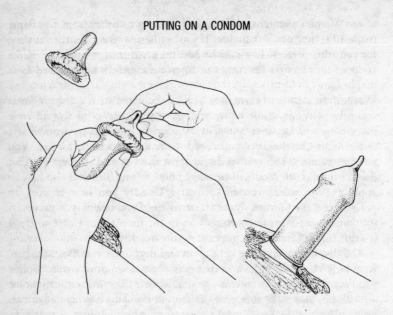

WHAT IT IS Simply, it's a rubber tube able to expand and fit on to the erect penis. There is often a teat on the end to collect the sperm. Condoms are usually lubricated, sometimes with a spermicide. Various brands are available, giving a choice of colours, some with ribs to increase vulval and vaginal stimulation, some specially flavoured. These can add to the fun, but to be safe they must be made to the British Standard specification (kite-marked) and used before their expiry date.

HOW IT WORKS By preventing sperm from entering the vagina.

FAILURE RATE 2–3 per cent, but can be better and also a lot worse depending on the user.

IS IT FOR YOU? As far as a woman is concerned it is free from side-effects and the responsibility belongs to the man. Some men and women develop an allergy to rubber (rare); special allergy condoms are available.

WHERE TO GET CONDOMS Condoms are available free from family planning clinics but not from your GP. You can buy them at the chemist, some supermarkets and petrol stations (check for the kite-mark, BSI), by mail order and from vending machines.

HOW TO USE A CONDOM The whole idea is that semen is kept within the condom, none is meant to escape. The teat end is pinched to get rid of any air and then the condom is rolled over the erect penis. Some women do this for their partner as part of love-making, but it must be done before there is any contact of the penis with the vulva. After ejaculation it's very important for the man to withdraw while the penis is still hard, holding on to the rim of the condom. This prevents any sperm leaking into the vagina. It isn't necessary to use a spermicide cream as well (some condoms come with spermicides in the rubber), but if you've had problems such as the condom breaking or slipping off, or if you have more than one partner, it may be a good idea. If you need extra lubrication use a water-based jelly (KY, not oil-based ones like Vaseline), or, better still, spermicidal jelly.

Only use a condom once and dispose of it in the bin.

Don't forget emergency contraception (page 80) if you have an accident (condom breaks or slips off).

ADVANTAGES The condom seems to protect the cervix from cervical cancer and CIN, and reduces the chances of getting sexually transmitted diseases, including HIV. It's free from side-effects and doesn't require you to be seen by a doctor. As far as sex goes, it can prolong intercourse by reducing the man's stimulation. This can help a woman to achieve her orgasm. There's no leaking or smell after intercourse either with a condom.

DISADVANTAGES AND SIDE-EFFECTS The big disadvantage of the condom is that it can interfere with the flow of intercourse and all the above advice may be forgotten. Some men complain about the decreased sensitivity and this can put them off. You do need to be meticulously careful every time for the condom to work.

REVERSIBILITY Barrier methods – diaphragm or condom – have no effect on your future fertility.

SPERMICIDES

WHAT THEY ARE These are usually antiseptic detergents – nonoxynol-9 and benzethonium – which kill sperm.

HOW THEY WORK Spermicides are inserted into the vagina as pessaries, foaming tablets, creams or aerosol foams. C-film is a small square of spermicide-impregnated material and is designed to be placed over the tip of the penis or over the entrance to the cervix. This is not a reliable form of contraception. Intercourse must take place within an hour of insertion of the spermicide. On their own they are not effective enough to protect against pregnancy.

FAILURE RATE Anything from 4 to 25 per cent; aerosol foams are

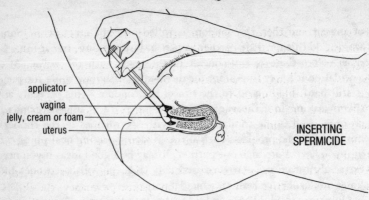

applicator
vagina
jelly, cream or foam
uterus

INSERTING SPERMICIDE

probably the most effective of these, the others are best used with additional methods.

WHERE TO GET SPERMICIDES From a chemist; they are also available from family planning clinics.

ADVANTAGES Spermicides are easily available over the counter, there are no health risks, the woman is in control, and there is some protection against sexually transmitted diseases (the detergent nonoxynol-9 is thought to kill HIV). They also provide some vaginal lubrication. They are very effective used with other methods — diaphragm, condom or IUD.

DISADVANTAGES AND SIDE-EFFECTS Some women are sensitive to spermicides, which make them sore and itchy. They are not a very reliable form of contraception.

REVERSIBILITY Spermicides have no effect on fertility.

THE SPONGE

WHAT IT IS A plastic disposable foam sponge (Today) impregnated with the spermicide nonoxynol-9.

HOW IT WORKS As a barrier method, the spermicide also kills sperm.

HOW TO USE THE SPONGE It is inserted high in the vagina after moistening it with tap water; it expands in the vagina. A small tape is attached so that it can be removed. The sponge can be put in well in advance of intercourse (up to twenty-four hours) and should be left in for at least six hours after the last intercourse. You don't need to use a new sponge if you have intercourse again during this twenty-four-hour period, but after that it must be thrown away.

FAILURE RATE This has quite a high failure rate, anything between 7 and 25 per cent.

IS IT FOR YOU? Not if you are sensitive to spermicides, and it's probably best not to use it while menstruating (risk of toxic shock syndrome). It is likely to be most appropriate for women who are less fertile (approaching the menopause or breastfeeding) and don't want to use any of the other methods.

WHERE TO GET THE SPONGE From a chemist; it is not available from family planning clinics.

ADVANTAGES It's easy to buy and use, and there's no need for extra spermicides.

DISADVANTAGES AND SIDE-EFFECTS As with spermicides alone, the sponge isn't effective enough protection against pregnancy; the Pill is twenty times more reliable. Some women (and men) have an allergic reaction to the spermicide, and it can be dislodged more easily than a diaphragm.

REVERSIBILITY Has no effect on fertility.

INJECTABLE CONTRACEPTION – *Depo-Provera*

Depo-Provera is licensed in the UK as a last-resort contraceptive only. This means it can only be considered by your doctor if it is not possible for you to use any other method or they are not acceptable to you. The other injectable available is Noristerat; it is usually offered for one-off use only (after a rubella vaccination or a vasectomy, for example).

WHAT IT IS A progestogen injection.

HOW IT WORKS By inhibiting ovulation and making the cervical mucus and the lining of the uterus unwelcoming to sperm.

WHERE TO GET IT From your doctor or family planning clinic.

HOW IT IS USED By injection in the buttocks. It must be renewed every twelve weeks.

IS IT FOR YOU? It is not recommended if you've just had a baby and are breastfeeding, or if you've just had a miscarriage or an abortion. Because fertility can be delayed for up to two years after stopping the injections, women should consider this carefully in case they might want children during this time. If you have cancer of the breast or of the reproductive organs, liver troubles, diabetes, arterial disease, or are already using regular medication for an illness, you should not choose Depo-Provera. The same applies to women who have weight problems or are suffering from depression.

FAILURE RATE Less than 1 per cent.

ADVANTAGES It's highly effective and requires no effort on the part of the woman once the injection has been given.

DISADVANTAGES AND SIDE-EFFECTS There is no way of reversing the effects of the injection once it has been given; the effects can last for anything up to ten months. It's important the woman clearly understands this. Her periods will probably become irregular and can even stop completely; this may last well after the injections are stopped, affecting fertility (see below). Other side-effects could be headaches, dizziness and mood changes. Some women experience either heavy or prolonged bleeding or both, which can lead to anaemia; sometimes this may go on for months after ceasing the injections. Depo-Provera lowers oestrogen levels, and can lead to periods stopping altogether. It has been linked to an increased risk of cancer in animals, although the evidence is not conclusive, and is certainly not suggestive in humans.

REVERSIBILITY It can take up to two years to get pregnant after stopping an injectable.

WHAT'S NEW

VAGINAL RING

This new contraceptive method works by releasing a small amount of progestogen every day, and will probably have an even better success rate than the Pill as there is nothing to remember.

The ring is made of silicone and is quite soft and squashy. It is inserted and sits at the top of the vagina, surrounding the cervix so periods come away as normal. It can stay in for three months.

It acts like the Mini-pill (page 67) to prevent pregnancy, but here the hormone is absorbed directly rather than being digested and broken down by the liver. This may reduce the side-effects.

Rings containing both oestrogen and a progestogen have also been developed; they are kept in for three weeks out of four. Both these rings can be taken out for a few hours with no loss of effectiveness.

THE FEMALE CONDOM

This is a disposable tube of polyurethane film with a closed tip (Femidom). It's held in place by flexible rings at one end around the cervix and the other around the labia. The success rate may be at least as good as the condom; it will also provide protection against sexually transmitted diseases. It does need practice to put in and can reduce sensitivity in the vulval area. Lubricating jelly must be used as there are no vaginal secretions.

HORMONAL IMPLANTS

These are capsules containing the hormone progestogen (Norplant), which are put under the skin in the arm. They can stay in for up to five years, releasing a small amount of hormone every day. There seems to be a very low failure rate, but in women weighing over 70 kg (10.5 stone) the failure rate appears to double. Like all the progestogen preparations it can affect your periods, and may share many of the side-effects of injectables (see opposite). Its advantage over the progestogen injection is that the capsules can be removed if necessary. It should be available within the next two years.

BACK TO NATURE

WITHDRAWAL (Coitus interruptus)

A very old method of contraception (mentioned in the Bible), in which the man withdraws his penis before ejaculation so that no sperm is deposited in the vagina. It's a method still commonly used in the developing world.

It's not the most effective form of contraception, but any contraception is better than none and in an emergency situation withdrawal is better than nothing. If it's your choice you can lower the risk of pregnancy by using a spermicide (pessary or sponge) as well (page 75).

ADVANTAGES It's free, no equipment is needed, and there are no side-effects.

DISADVANTAGES This is not a very effective method as sperm is sometimes released in semen before ejaculation. Intercourse can be unsatisfactory; a woman may feel anxious that her partner will not withdraw in time, the man may be anxious about this, too. This method doesn't provide any protection against sexually transmitted diseases, including HIV.

FAILURE RATE Difficult to gauge – one study claimed 8 per cent.

SYMPTO-THERMAL METHOD

This is based on avoiding intercourse at the time of ovulation.

FAILURE RATE Can be as low as 2 per cent and as high as 20 per cent.

IS IT FOR YOU? You must be prepared to think about your fertility every day, and have reasonably regular menstrual cycles. For this reason it's not suitable if you have irregular periods, have just had a baby or are coming up to the menopause. Your partner must understand the principles of the method and agree to abstinence from intercourse during your fertile phase (or use a condom). This may be difficult if you're not in a stable relationship.

WHAT IS INVOLVED You must take your temperature daily at the same time first thing in the morning using a special thermometer; check the vaginal secretions every evening, and possibly the position of the cervix, too; and work out your menstrual cycle over the previous year. Various signs indicate when you are ovulating: your temperature goes up (you can also get ovulation pain or a slight show of blood) and just before ovulation the cervical mucus becomes much heavier and more slippery: intercourse should be avoided until it becomes scanty again. Your individual fertile phase, usually of about eight to ten days, should also be calculated by looking at your periods over the last twelve months. Work out the shortest and longest cycles (the time from the beginning of one period to the beginning of the next). The following formula can then be used with the mucus appearance to work out your fertile phase. The shortest cycle (days) minus twenty gives the last infertile day. If your cycle was twenty-eight days, $28 - 20 = 8$. Your last infertile day is day eight. The longest cycle (days) minus eleven gives the last day of the fertile phase. If your longest cycle was thirty-two days, $32 - 11 = 21$. Your last fertile day is day twenty-one. You are therefore fertile between days eight and twenty-one.

Luteinising hormone (LH) surges just before ovulation and home kits are available to measure it. This may help to improve the accuracy of the sympto-thermal method.

This method requires some skill to work effectively; ideally, seek the help of a trained Natural Family Planning teacher.

DISADVANTAGES Doesn't provide any protection against venereal diseases, including HIV.

National Association of Natural Family Planning Teachers, 24 Selly Wick Drive, Selly Park, Birmingham B29 7JH. Tel: 021–472 3806.

EMERGENCY CONTRACEPTION

'MORNING-AFTER' PILL

Within three days of intercourse you can take a higher dose of the combined Pill (page 64) in two doses to prevent pregnancy. Go along to your doctor or family planning clinic as soon as you can. However, if you can't take the Pill for contraception then this method of emergency contraception won't be suitable for you.

The doctor will want to know when your last period was and when the unprotected sex took place. She will be very keen for you to get sorted out with a regular method of contraception. Two pills (either Eugynon or Ovran, each containing 50 micrograms of oestrogen) are taken straight away and two taken twelve hours later.

You may feel a little sick but if you vomit or have severe diarrhoea you will need some more pills. Your next period may be late.

The failure rate is about 1 per cent. It works by preventing either ovulation or stopping implantation if fertilisation has taken place.

FITTING AN IUD

This is an alternative to the 'morning-after' Pill and is suitable for up to five days after intercourse. If an egg has been fertilised then the IUD will prevent implantation in the uterus. The insertion is just like having an IUD fitted for contraception (page 68). However, for the same reasons, the IUD may not be a suitable form of long-term contraception for you; check with the doctor if it is safe to use in the circumstances. And if you don't want it as a future method of contraception it can be removed with the next period. There is a tiny failure rate.

Family Planning Association, 27–35 Mortimer Street, London W1N 7RJ. Tel: 071–636 7866.

PERMANENT SOLUTIONS

For a woman or a man, permanently abolishing fertility is a big step to take and the decision is best made after a period of thought and discussion. It's not a good idea to make your mind up at times of emotional stress, such as an unwanted pregnancy, after childbirth, or at the time of a divorce. More and more women, for example, are having to come to terms with divorce, often with young children. Remarriage is also becoming more common, and the desire to have more children with the new partner.

As a woman you must be clear in your own mind that you never want to be pregnant again, whatever happens.

STERILISATION FOR MEN: VASECTOMY

In a vasectomy the two tubes (the *vas deferens*) which carry the sperm from the testicles to the penis are cut. Sperm is still produced, but it is absorbed into the man's body instead of joining the seminal fluid. This can be done under a local anaesthetic, and usually takes less than half an hour. Afterwards, the man still produces semen and ejaculates after orgasm, but there is no sperm present. It may take three months before the last of the stored sperm has gone. Tests are done to check this (from masturbation specimens) but until the man gets the all-clear you must use another form of contraception. More than 50000 men have a vasectomy each year but recently scare stories have hit the press. Some American research has linked vasectomy with a higher incidence of kidney stones and prostate cancer in later life. As this is a common cancer in men over sixty-five anyway, it's not clear whether it would have developed with or without a vasectomy. There have been a number of reassuring studies that say there is no link.

REVERSAL It's easier to reverse a vasectomy than it is a female sterilisation, although this is still a delicate operation. The success rate at present is between 30 and 50 per cent, although fertility may be reduced.

VASECTOMY

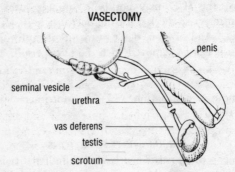

STERILISATION FOR WOMEN

In order to prevent pregnancy, each Fallopian tube is closed off so that sperm cannot reach the egg and the egg cannot move down to the sperm.

LAPAROSCOPIC CLIP STERILISATION The operation is done through a laparoscope via a small incision just below the navel (page 47). Through another small incision clips or rings are placed on the tubes which sterilises them; a very quick and simple method.

Some units make a small cut in the abdomen (*mini-laparotomy*) and either clip the tubes or cut and tie them. You usually stay in for a few days with this method.

Sterilisation does not cause weight gain or heavy periods.

Both these sterilisation techniques have very low failure rates of less than 0.5 per cent.

STERILISATION

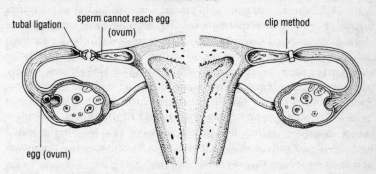

tubal ligation   sperm cannot reach egg   clip method
(ovum)

egg (ovum)

MYTHS AND MEN

There are a lot of old wives' tales about preventing pregnancy.

– Douching or washing the vagina after intercourse: sperm can be found in the cervix ninety seconds after ejaculation so it's got a headstart.

– Standing up during intercourse: the sperm are still deposited in the upper vagina near the cervix.

– Intercourse during a period: remember, sperm can live for four to five days. Some periods are not periods and can be the small bleed women occasionally get with ovulation.

– Stopping the penis going right in: intercourse and orgasm are both designed to encourage sperm up into the cervix and uterus so this can't work.

– Holding your breath: this must be quite difficult, but definitely a waste of time in terms of contraception.

– Jumping up and down afterwards: good exercise, maybe, but this won't stop those sperm well on their way into the cervix and uterus by the time you start jumping!

– Not having an orgasm: it is thought that orgasmic waves help sperm move up the Fallopian tubes, but they will still make it without an orgasm.

THE FUTURE

The search has been on for a male Pill for years. The difficulties with men are the large amount of sperm produced (200 million in every ejaculation), the three-month spell it takes to expel those already produced and stored in the testicles, and last, but certainly not least, worries about libido (women made very little fuss when the Pill was found to reduce desire). Weekly injections of testosterone have been promising but it's still very early days in terms of assessing its effectiveness.

In women vaccination against pregnancy using anti-human chorionic gonadotrophin (HCG, the hormone of pregnancy) is also being evaluated. This has some encouraging features: it appears to be cheap, reversible, long acting and with few side-effects.

SEXUALLY TRANSMITTED DISEASES

As the world population increases, with more people living in cities, and more people travelling and staying away from home, infections spread through sex have rocketed. At the same time, attitudes to sex have changed and the age of first intercourse has fallen. As a result, serious pelvic infection has risen by 50 per cent since the sixties; the major casualties are sexually active young teenagers and women in their early twenties.

Syphilis used to be the most serious problem, but it is rare these days. A far bigger concern today is chlamydia, which probably causes most infections in the Western world. Gonorrhoea, also rampant at one time, has been in decline since the mid-eighties. Herpes is still common and so is the virus that causes genital warts. Hepatitis B can be spread through sex as can the Human Immunodeficiency Virus (HIV) which eventually leads to AIDS.

THE GENITO-URINARY CLINIC

Some of the diseases that can be caught through sexual contact don't cause any symptoms. If you're in doubt find out from your doctor or local hospital where the nearest genito-urinary (GU) clinic is. Otherwise, try the local paper or telephone directory. Clinics call themselves genito-urinary medicine clinics, VD clinics or sexually transmitted diseases clinics, which can be confusing. It is best to go to one of these clinics if you think you have an infection as they specialise in these problems. The local hospital switchboard is probably the best way of finding out if you don't know.

What's a GU clinic like?

Most GU clinics are modern units often attached to the local hospital. They are open during hours to suit working men and women, with regular evening clinics. Often men and women are completely separated and have their own entrances and waiting rooms. The staff are usually sympathetic and helpful; it can be embarrassing to go to the clinic, but you are less likely to encounter disapproving attitudes nowadays, and you shouldn't be put off from seeking treatment.

On your first visit the doctor will want to know about your symptoms, your past sexual history and anything else that might be relevant. Details of your current partner will be necessary if you do have a sexually transmitted disease and he or she needs treatment.

You will be examined internally with a speculum (the same as for a cervical smear, page 30) and swabs taken from the cervix and vagina. A bimanual examination will check for any tenderness. Swabs may also be taken from the rectum and throat if you've been indulging in kissing or sucking your partner's penis or had anal intercourse. A blood and urine test should also be done.

The swabs are checked under the microscope there and then for an initial diagnosis, but cultures will also be grown to make sure this is accurate. You may be given treatment at your first visit or asked to come back for your results. It is very important that you do go back in case there is an infection; test results are usually not given over the telephone.

VAGINAL INFECTIONS

These are not sexually transmitted diseases but they can be investigated and treated at a GU clinic, or go to your own GP.

VAGINITIS AND VULVITIS

Vaginitis Every woman is aware that she produces secretions from the vagina. If the balance of good bacteria in the vagina is upset for some reason then the normal discharge becomes heavier and sometimes itchy. Some find this happens on the Pill or with an IUD fitted. Taking antibiotics, and allergies to perfumes or sprays applied to the vaginal area, can also make the discharge, and itching, worse. If this is a problem a little plain yogurt smeared just inside the vagina may help, as may adding some vinegar to the bath.

Any discharge that is irritating or smelly should be reported to the doctor (especially if you are sexually active).

Vulvitis If you are suffering from an itchy vulva – vulvitis – your doctor will need to check you for vaginal infection – thrush, warts, herpes, or infection elsewhere – scabies (tiny parasitic mites that burrow under the body skin) or threadworms in the anal area.

An allergy to a soap or perfume can cause a dermatitis as can a change in soap powder for the household washing.

Skin conditions like psoriasis can affect the vulva, as can diabetes. Sometimes the vulval skin becomes disordered, thin and weak in some parts and thickened and lumpy in others (*atrophic dermatoses*). Treatment can be difficult and steroid cream may be necessary if simple moisturising treatments (Eurax cream) don't work. It's best to get medical advice for this.

If you have trouble with vulval irritation go and see your doctor as soon as you can, there is usually a very simple solution, but it is always wise to make sure just in case.

Remember to keep the vulval area clean, washing daily with plain soap and water, wipe your bottom from front to back, wear cotton underwear and avoid feminine hygiene sprays and talcum powder in the crotch area.

THRUSH (*Candida albicans*)

This yeast infection is very common and once experienced is never forgotten. Candida naturally occurs in the vagina and bowel; it only causes problems when your body is out of balance for some reason and the yeast starts to grow. The symptoms include intense itchiness, especially at night, a feeling of soreness and a thick white discharge.

It is very common in pregnancy, when taking the Pill and in the second half of the cycle; sex can spark off an infection, as can antibiotics.

TREATMENT Pessaries work well (Canesten, Gyno-daktarin); sometimes you just need one pessary. Your doctor will usually want to take a swab first before prescribing treatment. Newer oral treatment (Sporanox) is now available.

PREVENTION Wash the vulval area carefully with soap and water every day, and avoid wearing tight trousers or underwear – try to keep the crotch area cool. Cotton underwear should be worn, not nylon.

BARTHOLIN'S ABSCESS

Bartholin's glands are the size of peas, one either side of the lower part of the vagina. Their secretions drain down a duct into the vagina. A gland gets infected from germs travelling up the duct (usually bowel organisms; it can also be gonorrhoea) and it becomes swollen, painful and red. Sitting down can be very uncomfortable. The gland fills up with pus like a large boil.

TREATMENT Surgical draining is often required if antibiotics have failed to clear up the infection.

SEXUALLY TRANSMITTED INFECTIONS

CHLAMYDIA TRACHOMATIS

This is a strange organism that seems to cause men a lot of trouble while women often don't know they've got it.

Chlamydia can live in the lining of the cervix for a long time causing no trouble. When it strikes it attacks the cervix, the tubes (pelvic inflammatory disease), the liver (*perihepatitis*) and sometimes the eyes (trachoma and eye infections).

Studies have looked at how common chlamydial infection is in the community – in one Scottish study as many as 12 per cent of women attending for a routine smear with no symptoms had definite chlamydia infection. Many of the other women had evidence that they had had an infection in the past.

Chlamydial infection can start as a severe pelvic infection with a high temperature and severe pain in the lower abdomen. You may or may not have a discharge, but intercourse is usually painful. Men get a sore urethra one to three weeks after contact, making it uncomfortable to urinate, as well as a discharge from the penis, and sometimes inflammation of the joints.

DIAGNOSIS This is usually made from genital swabs. If your doctor suspects chlamydia she may well go ahead and treat you while waiting for the results of the swabs.

TREATMENT Prompt antibiotics, usually of the tetracycline type, are necessary for at least ten days.

It is essential that both partners are treated. Unfortunately, untreated chlamydia can cause chronic pelvic pain and infertility.

TRICHOMONIASIS (TRICHOMONAS VAGINALIS)

Trichomonas vaginalis (also known as trich) is a one-celled parasite which causes vaginal itching, and is sometimes accompanied by a burning sensation; intercourse can be very sore. The discharge is frothy and smelly and can be white, green or brownish. The vulva can be reddened and mildly swollen.

Trichomoniasis is caught through sexual intercourse and can be passed from you to your partner and back again.

DIAGNOSIS A sample of the vaginal discharge is examined under the microscope.

TREATMENT A simple course of either metronidazole (Flagyl) or nimorazole (Naxogin) in tablet form is prescribed for you and your partner. It's best to avoid alcohol whilst taking them. Pessaries and vaginal treatment don't work. It's a good idea for you both to be fully checked out in case you have something else as well.

GONORRHOEA
In the same Scottish study mentioned above gonorrhoea was picked up in 1 per cent of women attending for a routine smear. Again, this is a silent infection in women, and 60 per cent can be infected for months without knowing. It, too, can cause inflammation of the Fallopian tubes as part of a pelvic infection, and can give a newborn baby an eye infection if the mother was infected.

Gonorrhoea is caused by the bacterium *gonococcus*, affecting the cervix, urethra, throat and anus. You can catch it from contact with the genitals and/or rectum of an infected person, including oral sex.

In the first few days after contact with an infected partner there can be difficulties with passing urine and sometimes a vaginal discharge. Not all women have these symptoms, probably only half of those infected. There is never a safe time when it comes to catching gonorrhoea, but the first half of the menstrual cycle is the time when infection in the tubes is more common. This gives the symptoms of acute pelvic infection with pain, temperature and discharge.

Men are usually sore at the tip of the penis and when passing urine but one in ten carry the infection without symptoms.

DIAGNOSIS If you suspect you have gonorrhoea or if your partner has symptoms you both need to be checked at your local GU clinic. There a swab will be taken for a culture test; it takes up to two days for the results to come through.

TREATMENT A penicillin-type of antibiotic is usually given and you should be called back for two negative culture tests to check the treatment has worked.

If you have multiple partners then there is a risk you may be harbouring gonorrhoea. Having regular checks at the GU clinic will detect it sooner. Better still, limit your number of partners and use a condom if in doubt. Beware if you see any discharge from your partner's penis or he complains of discomfort when passing urine.

GENITAL WARTS
These are caused by the *human papilloma virus* (HPV) and are spread by sexual contact; both men and women can have them. HPV loves the

warm moist areas in the vagina, around the anus and labia and on the cervix. The resulting warts can be very small or can be large growths like cauliflowers. Some types of the virus may have an effect on the development of cervical cancer so it's important to have warts treated.

DIAGNOSIS They're easy to see with the naked eye, except when they appear on the cervix. Then a colposcopy (page 32) will be necessary.

TREATMENT This usually involves applying a very strong liquid (podophyllin or trichloracetic acid) to the warts. Care must be taken as it burns normal skin. Very big warts or large numbers of them require cautery or laser treatment under general anaesthetic. How soon they clear up depends on how large they are.

Warts are contagious, so if you notice your partner has warts, or you have them, he must wear a condom. It's a good idea anyway if you're not sure about his previous sex life. A recent study has suggested that underwear could carry the virus and cause the return of warts, so wear fresh underwear every day.

HERPES

Herpes is caused by the *herpes simplex virus*, and both herpes simplex virus types can be responsible: HSV-1, the cold sore virus, can cause an attack of genital herpes by catching it from your partner's or from your own cold sores on the lips; HSV-2 is usually transmitted sexually. The first attack usually is the worst: small blisters on the vulva and vagina develop into painful sores with swelling. They take about a week to heal. You may feel generally unwell with fever and swollen glands. Further attacks are normally less severe and don't upset the whole system; the herpes effect is limited to the genitals. Many women never have more than one attack.

Herpes can only be transmitted when it is active – i.e. during an attack – so sex is out of the question if you are having an attack. Once the blisters are healed, sex is safe for you and your partner. If you have active herpes at the beginning of labour it could be a danger to the baby if born vaginally, so a caesarean section is usually recommended.

DIAGNOSIS The GU clinic will be able to diagnose whether you have herpes or not. During an attack, the sores are easy to see with the naked eye; however, a laboratory test will confirm this (usually a smear or a tissue culture).

TREATMENT Since a new drug (Acyclovir) has been developed, the treatment for herpes has been revolutionised. The drug, taken as tablets, stops the virus reproducing itself and this effect speeds up healing. The earlier the drug is given the better it will work. It is not recommended, however, for anyone with kidney or liver troubles.

Some women find their lives wrecked by frequent attacks of herpes and for them long-term Acyclovir treatment may be suggested. There's thought to be a stress element involved in bringing on repeated attacks, which may be when your general resistance is low.

Herpes has been linked to an increased risk of contracting cervical cancer, so regular smears are very important.

The Herpes Association, 41 North Road, London N7 9PD. They provide helpful information and a quarterly newsletter, *Sphere*.

SYPHILIS

Syphilis is caused by a spiral-shaped bacterium which gets into the body through tiny abrasions in the skin usually via the vulva or the cervix. It reproduces and after about a month forms a sore, usually on the vulva; this is known as *primary syphilis*. The sore is highly infectious but heals over after several weeks.

If no treatment is given, some weeks later a red pimply rash appears over the body which can last for as long as six weeks; this is *secondary stage syphilis*. Other symptoms can include inflamed joints, flu-like symptoms, sore throat, a sore in the mouth and loss of appetite.

The final stage, *tertiary syphilis*, may not appear until years later, and can result in skin ulcers, nervous complaints, blindness and heart and circulatory problems.

DIAGNOSIS A blood test at a GU clinic will show up the syphilis infection.

TREATMENT Syphilis is very easily treated with penicillin drugs by injection. Make sure you have two follow-up blood tests after treatment for an all-clear.

All pregnant women are tested for syphilis with a blood test as untreated it can be passed on to the baby and cause widespread fetal abnormalities.

PUBIC LICE (CRABS)

Pubic lice are similar to head lice but infest pubic hair. Crab-like in appearance, they are the size of a pinhead. They are caught mainly by sexual intercourse with an infected partner. They cause itching as the lice are bloodsuckers. Eggs (nits) are laid in the hairs and soon hatch into more lice.

TREATMENT Shampoos and lotions containing malathion are very effective; comb the pubic hair with a fine-tooth metal comb afterwards. You must make sure your partner is treated at the same time. If your skin is still itchy afterwards apply a soothing skin lotion.

MEN – SIGNS OF INFECTION TO LOOK OUT FOR
Beware if
– your partner complains of pain or difficulty in passing urine
– he has a discharge from the urethra at the tip of the penis
– he has any broken skin or sores in the genital area
– he has any skin irritation in the genital area
– you can see any warts on the penis, including the glans hidden by the foreskin.

HUMAN IMMUNODEFICIENCY VIRUS (HIV)
Infection with HIV can lead to Acquired Immune Deficiency Syndrome (AIDS), which means that the immune system is damaged. The disease was only discovered in 1981 but has already swept countries like Africa. In the United Kingdom 15000 people are known to be infected with HIV, 1500 of them women. These are people who have had the test for HIV, and there are probably many more with no idea that they are infected.

The at-risk groups are homosexual/bisexual men, injecting drug takers who share needles, people who have received infected blood or blood products, and all the sexual partners of these people. In this country most infected people are homosexual men. In parts of Africa, South America and the Caribbean, however, the spread is by heterosexual sex, and as many women as men are affected. HIV seems bound to spread into the heterosexual community here and latest figures (1990) indicate that about a third of new cases in Scotland and a sixth of new cases in England are women.

How is the virus caught?
HIV is very fragile and cannot survive outside the body. It is present in all body fluids in an infected person, but only blood, semen and vaginal secretions have enough of the virus to be infectious. Even then, relationships exist where one partner is HIV positive and the other is not, so it would seem that it is possible to come into sexual contact with an infected person without catching it. However, it also seems clear that the more you come into contact with the virus, the more

likely you are to become infected with HIV.

It can be transmitted through vaginal or anal sex. If there are any cuts, tears or ulcers in the vagina, infected semen can easily be absorbed; it can also be absorbed through the vaginal lining even where there is no damage. It's easier, therefore, for a woman to catch HIV than a man in heterosexual sex, because the pool of semen stays in the vagina for much longer than the vaginal secretions stay on a man's penis. Anal sex can result in small tears in the anal wall, again making transmission easier.

If either partner suffers from bleeding gums, mouth ulcers or sores, oral sex can be risky. And because the lining of the mouth is a mucous membrane (like the vagina), this could be another route for the virus.

Sharing needles with an infected person can pass the virus on. This has led to a high rate of infection in drug users who inject themselves.

What are safe activities?

It isn't thought that saliva can transmit the virus, so kissing closed and open mouthed is considered safe, and you can't catch HIV from sharing cups or towels.

You can't get the virus from holding hands or cuddling an infected person. The virus can only pass into the body if there is a break in the skin.

You can't get the virus from a swimming pool or public toilet.

Blood for transfusion and Factor 8 for haemophiliacs is now screened for HIV virus and is safe.

Dentists use disposable needles and proper sterilisation techniques.

What does the virus do?

Once HIV enters the blood stream the virus attacks the white blood cells that protect the body from infection (the immune system). The body reacts by producing antibodies, which can keep the virus in check for a limited time, but doesn't destroy it completely. Some people have a flu-like illness while the antibodies are being produced: feeling tired, with a headache and a high temperature. (Note: these symptoms are very common with many infections.) AIDS itself may not develop for years (the current figures suggest 39 per cent of people will develop AIDS within nine years of infection with HIV). It seems likely that anyone infected with HIV will go on to have AIDS in time.

AIDS itself means the immune system is attacked. Symptoms can be loss of weight, night sweats and fever. Lowered resistance of the immune system can leave the way open for normally rare conditions, including widespread thrush, tuberculosis and a type of pneumonia called *Pneumocystis carinii*. A rare skin cancer (*Kaposi's sarcoma*) develops in a quarter of AIDS cases. Women may face an increased risk of cancer of the cervix, herpes infection, genital ulceration and tuberculosis of the pelvis.

Women infected with HIV face a 15–33 per cent chance of infecting their unborn child. This would be acceptable grounds for terminating the pregnancy. If the pregnancy goes ahead fetal growth seems to be unaffected. It is possible that pregnancy in an HIV-positive woman may bring on AIDS itself more rapidly.

Diagnosis and treatment

If you have been infected with HIV the antibody reaction usually takes up to three months to develop and show up in the blood. This can, however, be as soon as six weeks and take as long as nine months. If you think you have caught HIV you can have a blood test which tests for these antibodies. Depending on when you think you could have been infected a three-month waiting period is recommended.

Most people go to a GU clinic or their family doctor for the test; this is absolutely confidential. You must think long and hard, however, about the consequences of a positive test before you have one, the effect on your life, and, if you are in a relationship, your partner's life; pregnancy and infection; as well as practical considerations, such as insurance problems.

TREATMENT There is no cure for AIDS at present. The drug AZT (Zidovudine) can slow down the progression of the disease and so possibly prolong life.

Drug companies are focusing their resources on finding a vaccination against HIV and a cure for AIDS, but no solutions have been found yet.

How to live more safely

Use a condom if there is any doubt about you or your partner's past, together with a spermicidal cream containing nonoxynol-9 (this acts as a germicide for the virus). Used properly, condoms can cut down the risk of catching HIV by 90 per cent. Anal intercourse is risky; if you do it then use a condom. Oral sex is thought to be safe if there are no breaks in the skin in the mouth or on the genitals, but this is not always easy to see.

Masturbation by yourself or with your partner is fine as long as semen doesn't go anywhere near the vaginal area. Kissing, stroking and hugging each other are all safe activities.

Don't share needles or syringes if you inject drugs, and beware of dirty needles and instruments used for tattoos and ear piercing in the back streets.

The future
Apparently, most new infections in the USA are in the fifteen–nineteen-year-old age group. AIDS is the leading cause of death for women aged between twenty and forty in America and in some parts of Africa.

Sadly, the UK appears to be going the same way. A recent study in the UK suggested that a quarter of all fourteen-year-olds have had sex already. It is vital, therefore, that our children understand about safe sex, and that young girls have the courage and confidence to insist on a condom (hard enough for anyone in a new relationship). The realistic way for schools and parents to protect our children, therefore, is to provide practical, realistic sex education.

National Aids Helpline. Tel: 0800 567123. A 24-hour service with advice and information.
Terence Higgins Trust, 52–4 Gray's Inn Road, London WC1 8JU. Tel: 071–242 1010. Offers support, counselling and help for anyone worried about AIDS or HIV infection.
AVERT (AIDS Education and Research Trust), PO Box 91, Horsham, W. Sussex RH13 7YR. Send an s.a.e for helpful booklets on AIDS.

UNWANTED PREGNANCY
If you think you could be pregnant and you don't want to be, the best thing you can do first is to get it confirmed. A pregnancy test kit bought from the chemist is extremely accurate and sensitive; it can pick up a pregnancy on the day you miss a period. If it's positive, you may experience a whole range of feelings, from being too scared to tell your family because of how they may react, not sure what to do, and feeling alone and vulnerable, to fear about becoming a mother, and anger that this has happened to you. The options you may want to consider at this stage are keeping the baby, continuing with the pregnancy and having the baby adopted, or terminating the pregancy. These can be very difficult decisions to make for some women, and getting as much help and support as possible are essential to cope with the problem.

If you decide to keep the baby, it helps to have someone to support you with this, such as a husband, boyfriend or mother. But make sure you are doing what you want, not what everyone else wants.

Adoption is urged on some mothers-to-be, but there are women who have deeply regretted this decision later on. You are looked after in pregnancy just like any mother, and at delivery you can see and care for the baby if you like. You can also change your mind at any time about adoption. If you can go through with it you will be making an infertile couple somewhere extremely happy.

Deciding whether to have an abortion can bring up a whole mixture of feelings: whether you will regret later on not going ahead and having the baby, feelings of fear about the abortion itself, whether you'll ever be able to enjoy sex and a relationship with a man again, for example. Most women who have had an abortion reported afterwards that they felt they had made the right decision, although that didn't stop them feeling sad. Many of them had the support of a good friend, family members or a partner during the whole experience; if you can, find someone to be with you and help you through this difficult time.

TERMINATION OF PREGNANCY

If you think you want an abortion, first go and see your own doctor and discuss it with her. There's a good chance that she will support you whatever your decision. If you have already definitely decided to have an abortion, tell her this on your first visit. If it's obvious from her reaction that she will not help you she may refer you to another family doctor, or you could try one of the big charities such as the Pregnancy Advisory Service (PAS, London only) or the British Pregnancy Advisory Service (BPAS).

Assuming your doctor is sympathetic, she should counsel you, giving you any information and advice you need. Before a termination can be done an abortion form must be signed by two doctors stating the reason for doing it. These include severe abnormalities of the fetus, danger to the mother's life, and harm to existing children if the pregnancy continued. Most 'social' abortions are done to prevent deterioration in the mother's mental health.

Your doctor will make the hospital appointment for you, and the hospital should come back to you within a week with the date and time of your appointment. If there is any problem with a waiting list, especially if it puts you over twelve weeks pregnant, you may want to consider going to one of the charities mentioned above. There is a charge, however, for these terminations.

SUCTION (VACUUM) ABORTION (UP TO 13 WEEKS)

This technique is similar to a D & C (page 50) in that, under a general anaesthetic, the cervix is first stretched gently with graduated metal rods. A suction tube (curette) is then put into the inside of the uterus and the fetus and placenta sucked out. This technique is quick, clean and safe. It can be done as a day case, although some units like you to stay in for a night or two.

RISKS Perforation of the uterus: a pregnant uterus is soft and even with care a hole may be made in the uterus. This may need surgery to repair it, or just antibiotics and observation.

Retained fetal tissue: it can be difficult sometimes to make sure everything has been removed. Bleeding and infection can follow in the days and weeks after. This needs prompt attention, with antibiotics and another trip to the hospital or clinic to remove any remaining tissue. If untreated, the infection can travel to the Fallopian tubes and cause damage and possibly infertility.

Cervical incompetence: the cervix may be damaged during dilatation, affecting its ability to hold in a subsequent pregnancy, leading to late miscarriages and premature labour.

Afterwards you may have some pain and strong cramps and feel shaky and nauseous. If you are a day case, you can sit or lie down in a recovery room before going home.

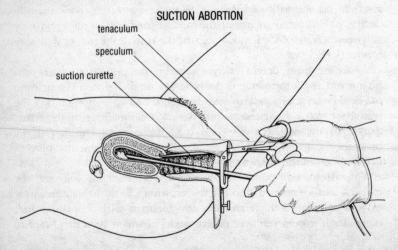

SUCTION ABORTION

tenaculum

speculum

suction curette

MID-TRIMESTER ABORTION (AFTER 12 WEEKS)

Abortions can now be carried out up till twenty-four weeks gestation. In practice most gynaecologists are unhappy to consider terminating pregnancies beyond twenty weeks.

As the fetal parts are bigger the technique for mid-trimester abortion is different. Prostaglandins are used to induce labour either by inserting pessaries, or through a tube gently placed inside the cervix. You are wide awake throughout. An intravenous drip with syntocinon helps the uterus to contract, and the fetus is usually passed within twenty-four hours. Often the placenta is stuck and needs to be removed surgically under a general anaesthetic. The procedure can be painful and the nursing staff will give pain relief when needed. It is certainly much more of an ordeal physically and emotionally than an early termination, since you experience labour and may see a recognisable fetus when it's over. This can be especially hard for women who are having an abortion following tests for fetal abnormality. The loss can be akin to stillbirth or neo-natal death (page 140), and they may need special counselling to help them through what is for many a devastating experience. You need to be in hospital for at least two nights.

RISKS These are similar to those of an early abortion (see opposite), but are slightly higher.

After the abortion

Bleeding settles down within a week and a period follows four to six weeks later. If necessary, contraception is discussed and sorted out before you are discharged from hospital.

Many women feel bewildered, confused and very guilty afterwards. A grief reaction can set in which can be prolonged if support and sympathy are not available. If you're finding it difficult to come to terms with an abortion and feel you can't tell anyone, talk to your family doctor, who knows exactly what's happened. A counselling service may be available.

What's new

RU 486 (mifeprostone) is a 'designer' drug specially developed to act against the hormone progesterone. It looks set to revolutionise abortion methods in this country. It's been approved for use from summer 1991, but it will take a while for doctors to familiarise themselves with the drug and work out the best way of using it within the hospital. It is used in France for women wanting an early abortion before seven weeks; that is, when the period is three weeks late.

Up to the seventh week a pregnancy needs progesterone from the ovary to keep it going, after that the placenta produces enough of its own. If the progesterone is blocked early on the pregnancy will fail.

Trials have shown that prostaglandins must be taken, by injection or pessary, two days after the RU 486 to make it reliably effective. You pass the fetus three to four hours after the prostaglandin treatment, usually under supervision in hospital; surgery is hardly every required. No overnight stay is necessary, but some women may find actually miscarrying themselves rather than a termination under general anaesthetic more distressing.

RU 486 is currently under investigation as a method of birth control, as emergency contraception and for inducing labour.

Old wives' tales

If you're scared you're pregnant you may feel you'd try anything to bring your period on. Home remedies don't work: gin and hot baths and caster oil will only make you feel dreadful, they will not bring on an abortion. The same applies to jumping from a height. Dirty instruments or knitting needles inserted into the uterus cause pelvic infection, bleeding, infertility and death.

With today's more relaxed and tolerant attitudes to abortion, women should know that they will have sympathetic treatment and counselling from their local family doctor and consultant.

RAPE AND VIOLENCE

Being raped or indecently assaulted is most women's nightmare. Rape is defined in British law as sexual intercourse without a woman's consent. This may or may not involve ejaculation or physical violence. Indecent assault is any other form of sexual attack, which includes putting foreign bodies into the vagina, anal or oral sex. It is a traumatic event that can happen to women of all ages and backgrounds. We need to know how to avoid it, how to stop it if possible if it's happening, and what to do if it's happened to you.

Avoiding rape

In quite a large proportion of rapes the attacker is known to the victim, many are planned and more than half happen indoors, often in the woman's own home. It's now been accepted in law that rape can happen within marriage. Rapists have a wide range of characteristics, but commonly they have been violent before and many are drunk (rapists who kill their victims are rare). This is the same profile as for other violent crimes, suggesting that rape has more to do with violence than sex itself.

Make sure you have good locks on the doors and windows at home. On the street, avoid known trouble spots, and if you are walking try not to go home around closing time (50 per cent of rapists are drunk when they attack). If you have a car, never leave it unlocked, and try to park it near a street light at night. Look into the back seat before getting in. You may want to take some self-defence classes.

Stopping rape
Try to keep your cool. Make a decision whether or not it's possible to escape. If it is, aim for the groin or upper abdomen with your knee or fist and really mean it. A Home Office study suggests that the sooner you act aggressively, the more likely you are to avoid rape. But in the end do anything you feel is right to ensure you survive.

It's happened – what next?
Women who have been raped will feel dirty, ashamed, abused and deeply shocked; it is important to call a girlfriend or relative or the local rape crisis centre for comfort and support.

To press charges against the rapist the police must be informed as soon as possible: don't wash or change your clothes (even though you may desperately want to), avoid drinking any alcohol, and try to remember the sequence of events leading up to the rape including a description of the rapist.

See a doctor as soon as possible to check for any sexually transmitted diseases, and you may want to take a 'morning-after' Pill if there is a chance you could be pregnant (page 80).

Counselling can help you cope with the immediate and long-term effects of rape. Some women find difficulties in establishing a normal relationship again and need help.

Rape Crisis Centre, PO Box 69, London WC1. Tel: 071–837 1600. Offers counselling help and support.
Women's Aid National Helpline. Tel: 0272 633542. Helpful if you're experiencing violence in the home.

—4—
PREGNANCY AND BIRTH

Having a baby can mean one of the biggest upheavals in a woman's life. Being responsible for another human twenty-four hours a day takes quite a bit of getting used to, and you will need energy and strength that you never thought you had. You may also experience intense physical and emotional bonding with your newborn baby. For some it can be a wonderful experience, despite the hard work, for others the baby may seem a burden, a source of constant anxiety, and they may feel housebound and very isolated. Having a baby means changing your relationships with your partner, family and friends. This can take a period of adjustment while you and your partner get used to the baby and your new roles; if there are already problems in the relationship, however, a child will not necessarily help – it can add more stress as well as money worries.

GETTING FIT FOR A BABY
Getting yourself and your partner in the best condition *before* you get pregnant gives the baby the best chance of being healthy.

TOXINS Give up poisons, such as tobacco and alcohol. The odd drink doesn't seem to do any harm, but chronic alcohol abuse and nights of heavy binge drinking affect sperm production and cause problems with fetal development (see Women and Alcohol, page 14). Smoking also affects sperm, which means there are more unsuccessful pregnancies overall (see Women and Smoking, page 15), so you should stop now and forever; smoking in pregnancy means that the fetus does not grow so well. If you drink lots of coffee too, you should try to cut down.

You should both avoid unnecessary drugs; tell your doctor if you're trying for a baby.

Avoid any dangers at work such as exposure to X-rays, or dangerous chemicals. For example, 2,4,5–T, a pesticide, contains dioxin, a poisonous chemical which has been linked with miscarriages and birth defects. Some flea sprays contain toxic substances, as does wood preservative. Exposure to lead also affects fertility in both men and women, including malformed sperm, miscarriage and birth defects. Working with visual display units isn't thought to cause any problems.

DIET Follow a good diet with plenty of fresh fruit and vegetables, which is high in fibre and low in fat (page 11). Try to take regular exercise (page 12).

BLOOD TESTS It is a good idea to check you are immune to German measles (rubella). You will need a blood test from your GP. Rubella causes most damage to the baby in the first three months of pregnancy and once you're pregnant you can't be vaccinated.

You may also want the doctor to check for anaemia and, if you are Rhesus negative, Rhesus antibodies (page 109).

SEXUALLY TRANSMITTED DISEASES If you have any reason to suspect you are infected, get a check-up and treatment.

PETS If you have pets, be extra careful about hygiene. Remember to wash your hands after handling them and if possible get your partner to change the cat litter tray if you have one. *Toxoplasmosis* germs are carried in cats' faeces and raw or undercooked meat and the infection can be passed to the fetus. It can cause miscarriage or, if the pregnancy continues, brain and blood problems in the baby.

PRE-PREGNANCY CLINIC SERVICE Some hospitals and family doctors now offer this service; it is particularly helpful for women who suffer from chronic diseases or conditions such as diabetes, who have a slightly higher risk of fetal abnormality. Epileptic women and those taking long-term drugs need to know what effect these will have on the baby.

The pre-pregnancy clinic may also offer genetic counselling; if not, you may be advised by your GP to see a genetic counsellor if you or your partner fall into any one of the following categories:

– if a close relative suffers from a disabling disease

– couples who have already had a child with a birth defect or a child who has inherited a genetic disease

– women who have already had two or more stillbirths or miscarriages

– African or Caribbean couples, to check for sickle-cell trait and sickle-cell anaemia (page 110)

– couples of Mediterranean, Middle Eastern, Indian or Pakistan origin, to check for thalassaemia, a similar blood disorder to sickle-cell anaemia (page 110)

– Eastern European Jews, to check for Tay-Sachs disease, a fatal condition affecting the nervous system.

How long will it take to get pregnant?

If you and your partner are both healthy and in your twenties, it should take between three and six months after stopping birth control, but up to a year is considered normal. It can take longer for a woman over thirty (page 107), especially if her partner is over thirty too.

HEALTH CARE DURING PREGNANCY

Getting pregnant can be quite a shock to the system, and from the moment your period is late, a number of changes are swinging into action. For a start you may notice you are urinating more often, your breasts feel tender, and some foods and substances make you feel nauseated. You may also feel more tired than normal.

PREGNANCY TEST A sensitive pregnancy test (measuring *human chorionic gonadotrophin*, HCG, the hormone found in the urine of pregnant women) is available from the chemist and can usually give a result the same day your period is due (a sample of urine taken at any time of day will do).

Your doctor or family planning clinic can also arrange a pregnancy test (latex) at the local hospital, but this actually may not be such a sensitive test. This is done after your period is two weeks late and requires a specimen of the first urine passed in the morning. Take it along to your doctor in a clean bottle. If you can't wait to find out, buy an HCG test from the chemist and do it yourself. However, they are quite expensive and care must be taken to follow the instructions to the letter. If this is positive, have another test done by your doctor when you're two weeks late. She will not necessarily want to examine you, but she will want to know if you've had any symptoms of bleeding or pain (early signs of threatened miscarriage – page 115 – or ectopic pregnancy – page 118). It's not easy to confirm a pregnancy by examination until you are eight or ten weeks on from your last period. Your doctor will arrange a hospital appointment to register the pregnancy; this is called the booking visit.

ESTIMATED DATE OF DELIVERY (EDD) This can be calculated by working out the date of your last menstrual period and adding on nine months and seven days. For example, if your last period started on 15.8.92 then the baby would be due on 22.5.93. However, if your periods are irregular or you've just come off the Pill, the date of your last period may not be an accurate guide to your delivery date. Where this is the case, ultrasound scanning (page 112) before twenty-four weeks can provide a fairly accurate date.

ANTE-NATAL CARE

Most women sail through their pregnancies with no problems at all. But for a few, trouble arises quite unpredictably. Early detection of problems can avoid serious situations happening later that may affect both the mother and the baby's life. The tests to look for fetal abnormalities are done before twenty weeks so it's vital that women who may be at risk come to the clinic well in advance.

At the hospital booking visit the midwife will take your medical details, check your weight and blood pressure, and take blood and urine samples. You will also have a general physical examination. You can discuss with the midwife the sort of birth you want at this first visit (page 124), and she will book you in if you are having the baby in hospital. After that, the visits are shorter. These entail checking the size of the baby and listening to the fetal heart, checking your weight and blood pressure and a urine test. This is the time to air anything else that's worrying you, and to discuss the birth itself: what sort of pain relief you want, what view the hospital takes on active birth, and so on. Usually the hospital and the family doctor will share your ante-natal care. If you are having a normal straightforward pregnancy your doctor will do most of it, if there are problems the hospital consultant or junior staff will see you more often. Many women with normal pregnancies are looked after almost entirely by midwives.

Ante-natal visits are usually monthly until you are twenty-eight weeks pregnant, every two weeks until thirty-six weeks and then weekly until you have the baby. You'll be given a cooperation card which records your results and your progress in the pregnancy. Carry it with you until you have the baby. It contains vital information which may be invaluable if problems arise when you're away from home.

EATING IN PREGNANCY

Doctors take a much more relaxed view of weight gain in pregnancy these days. Your weight is checked at each ante-natal visit: too much may mean there may be excessive swelling, too little may mean the baby isn't growing well enough. Usually, most women gain between 7 and 14 kg (15 to 30 lb) gradually throughout the pregnancy. About a quarter of this total is put on in the first twenty weeks, a half between twenty and thirty weeks and the rest in the last ten weeks. Everyone is different, though. This is definitely not the time to start slimming, but if you're worried about your weight discuss this at the clinic.

A healthy mother equals a healthy baby, so a good diet is even more important when you're planning a pregnancy or are actually pregnant. What is a good diet? Here's a *rough guide* to a balanced day's diet:

1. Fish, meat, eggs, pulses, nuts – two helpings
2. Fruit and vegetables – four helpings
3. Milk, cheese, yogurt – three helpings
4. Bread, rice, pasta, cereals – three helpings.

This is a basic guide and includes all the necessary protein, fats and carbohydrates. Whenever possible use fresh food, especially fresh fruit and vegetables. To help supply your roughage choose wholemeal bread, brown rice and wholemeal pasta, especially if you are having problems with constipation. Avoid caffeine – coffee, tea, chocolate. An excess of caffeine-type stimulants may have a disturbing effect on the fetus; recent research suggests that the combined effects of smoking, alcohol and coffee drinking makes babies smaller.

Listeria This bacterial infection has recently been found to cause miscarriages and stillbirths. The affected mothers have had a flu-like infection only.

The bacteria live in the soil and in animal faeces and can thrive in uncooked meats, unwashed vegetables and unpasteurised milk. For this reason, it's best not to eat cheese made from unpasteurised milk, pâtés, uncooked meats and ready prepared salads. Listeria bacteria can multiply in temperatures below 7°C but are killed if food is thoroughly cooked to 70°C. All meat and all prepared meat dishes kept in the fridge must be cooked very carefully; microwave instructions should be followed exactly.

SEX AND EXERCISE

Sex There's no harm in continuing to make love once you are pregnant. But things are different: you may feel particularly turned on in the early months, your nipples and clitoris may feel that bit more sensitive and having an orgasm may be easier and better. On the other hand, if you feel sick all the time, or extremely tired, sex will be the last thing on your mind (this should get better as the pregnancy progresses, however).

Your partner is also noticing the changes, and while some men are turned on by pregnancy, others find it the complete reverse. Some women feel most unattractive, fat, cumbersome and definitely unsexy throughout their pregnancy. Whatever the case, it's important to reassure each other of still being loved and wanted.

As you get bigger it can become more awkward making love with the man on top. Change positions to side or rear entry or with the woman on top. (The baby is well away from the activity, positioned above the cervix cushioned in a bag of fluid.) Don't forget to show affection in other ways, such as kissing and cuddling, when sex isn't right for you. If there is a problem, talk about it. Tell him if you feel unattractive and unloved, or if you'd rather have a rest from sex — let him know rather than build up resentment. There are plenty of things to think about with the new baby coming without relationship worries.

The only time you may want to abstain from having sex in the early stages of pregnancy is if you've had a miscarriage before. In such cases, perhaps it is a good idea to abstain for the first twelve weeks. No one has ever proved that sex can cause a miscarriage, but couples may feel this is the one thing they can do something about. If you've had any bleeding it's best to take advice from your doctor.

Exercise Even if you're fit and take regular exercise, you must be cautious in pregnancy. As the demands of the fetus increase on your system, strenuous exercise can divert some of the blood destined for the placenta to the muscles of your arms and legs and general circulation. It's best, therefore, to convert the more active exercise like running and aerobics to gentle jogging and swimming. Stop when you are tired, and don't push yourself to achieve targets, such as a certain number of lengths. If the uterus starts tightening, it's definitely time to slow down.

CLASSES IN COPING

Parentcraft classes will be taking place at your local hospital or National Childbirth Trust (NCT) group. Hospital classes usually start in the sixth or seventh month of pregnancy so that it's all fresh in your mind when the baby arrives. Partners are very welcome.

The classes aim to increase your understanding of the childbirth process so that you go into labour with confidence and in control. Knowing what to expect in terms of the contraction pains, the stages of labour and what happens along the way really will help to make the whole thing relaxed and even enjoyable. Your partner, too, will be able to be that much more supportive if he's not intimidated by the staff and surroundings and knows what's going on.

You will learn deep breathing and relaxation exercises to help with the contractions in labour, as well as other exercises, including the essential pelvic floor exercises (page 150).

Parentcraft will also help teach you about the new baby: what to expect in the baby's development, how to cope with feeding — in fact a good general idea of what it's all going to be about.

MATERNITY BENEFITS

More and more women carry on working while they are pregnant. Many even delay starting a family until their thirties in order to develop a career before a break.

Pregnant women are entitled to eighteen weeks paid maternity leave if they have been working for the same employer for at least forty-one weeks before the birth, have paid National Insurance for at least eight weeks during this time, and if they stay at work until eleven weeks before the birth.

If you have been in the job for two years, you are then entitled to six weeks on pay-related earnings plus twelve weeks at the standard rate. This also entitles you to job security providing you have informed your employer, *in writing*, and least twenty-one days before leaving, that you are going on maternity leave and plan to return to work afterwards. This entitles you to leave of eleven weeks before and twenty-nine weeks after the birth. Again, twenty-one days before returning to work, you must let your employer know, *in writing*, that you are returning to work. Or if your employer writes to you about this, you must respond, *in writing*, within fourteen days of getting a letter.

Leaflets available from the clinic will tell you all about other benefits. Some pregnant women are entitled to free milk and vitamins (contact your local benefit office); all women are entitled to free prescriptions and free dental treatment until a year after the birth (get the correct form from your doctor or the clinic). It's a good idea to take advantage of the free dental treatment, as your gums need special care during pregnancy. A maternity grant is also available if you or your partner is receiving income support or family credit. A state maternity allowance scheme is available for self-employed women, or if you have changed employers, or left work early. Claim forms are available from Social Security offices or the post office. You should be allowed time off within working hours to attend for ante-natal visits.

Working and being pregnant can be exhausting. The morning rush, fighting traffic or commuters, may be hard to cope with, especially if you are feeling sick in the early months. Try to change your hours and leave earlier or later. If you have a partner, involve him more with the housework and shopping at this stage, and relax — let things slide for the time being, you can always catch up later. If you are on your own, call on your family and/or friends and accept all offers of help. You can feel especially alone and vunerable at this time, and you will need all the support you can get. A French study has shown that the chances of premature labour increase the more strenuous and arduous the work.

Doctors have looked at the birth weight of babies of working and non-working mothers and found that it doesn't seem to make any difference whether you work or not.

PREGNANCY AND THE OLDER WOMAN

There are basically three kinds of women who delay childbearing into their thirties.

Career women Committed to long professional training with a climb up the career ladder, these are normally low-risk women. Well paid, well nourished and well informed on health matters, they usually have very few problems in pregnancy.

Infertile couples Not a deliberate delay, but a pregnancy can follow years of treatment and anxiety, or where there may have been problems such as disordered hormones or fibroids. The chances of having a healthy baby once the early problems have been dealt with, are as good as the next woman.

Single women It may not be until you are over thirty that you meet the man for you. Unfortunately, you can't do a great deal about this, but in the meantime keep fit and healthy.

Getting pregnant in your thirties may not be as easy as it would have been in your twenties. Several studies have shown that thirty-one is the critical age, after which your chances of conceiving do start to fall. This seems to be due to a gradual deterioration in the quality of the eggs, but your partner's fertility is also decreasing as he gets older. (If you should have difficulties in conceiving, it is usually best for you both to be tested for any fertility problems – page 141). Women in their thirties, therefore, usually take longer to get pregnant. The over-thirties also have more miscarriages. Again, this is probably related to the quality of the egg.

Problems in later pregnancy are more common, too. Older women are more likely to have fibroids (page 56), which sometimes cause miscarriage or obstruction in labour. There is an increased risk of high blood pressure (which can affect the amount of oxygen the baby is getting, or be a sign of pre-eclampsia, page 122) and premature labour.

The chances of ending up with a caesarean section (page 138) are higher for the woman over thirty-five expecting her first baby than for a younger woman. Perhaps the subtle influence that there isn't much time left, and that there are fewer chances of conceiving before the menopause, has some effect on the woman and the doctor who is looking after her. If there's a decision to be made about delivery, the mother's age may just swing it over to caesarean section.

Chromosome abnormalities increase with maternal age (for example, the older you get the greater the risk of having a baby affected with Down's syndrome), but these can be easily tested for using the early technique of CVS (page 110) or the later amniocentesis (page 111). It's important in such cases to consider beforehand whether you would have the pregnancy terminated if Down's is diagnosed. There is a slight chance of miscarriage with these tests, and you may have already decided you want to keep the baby.

GENERAL ADVICE Don't be put off having a baby because of your age, but follow the good health guidelines for pregnancy – a well-balanced diet, no smoking, no alcohol – and, very importantly, get ante-natal care as early as possible.

GROWING A BABY

The sperm joins the egg in the Fallopian tube. The fertilised egg then divides several times and travels down to the uterus to implant about five days later. Non-identical twins are the result of two eggs being released by the ovary, which are then fertilised by two separate sperms. Identical twins occur when the fertilised egg splits into two. The sperm determines the sex of the baby and carries either an X chromosome for a girl or a Y chromosome for a boy. This joins the mother's X chromosome in the egg. The bundle of cells grown from the fertilised egg divide into an embryo part and a placenta part in the uterus. At forty weeks there is a placenta and a fully formed fetus lying in a bag of amniotic fluid.

The placenta is attached to the lining of the uterus and to the umbilical cord. It filters blood from the mother so that oxygen and nutrients are carried down the umbilical cord to the baby. Waste from the baby is carried back and filtered into the mother's blood circulation. The placenta is vital – things that damage the placenta damage the baby. Smoking and high blood pressure, for example, can lead to small babies and the risk of fetal distress.

Amniotic fluid, contained in the amniotic sac, is another essential. It enables the baby to swim around in a constant temperature, practise breathing movements, and cushions her from any bumps on the mother's abdomen. The baby swallows the fluid and also urinates into it. A shortage of fluid can suggest that the placenta is not working properly and the baby's growth is slow.

TESTS DURING PREGNANCY

In the first three months all the baby's organs develop, so it's a critical time for everything to go well. That's why it's important for a woman trying for a baby to be fit and well in those early weeks before she knows she is pregnant.

At the hospital booking visit (page 103) you may be offered certain tests for fetal abnormalities, depending on your age and family history. Don't be rushed into making decisions about these: some have complications. They are not for you if you could never agree to terminating the pregnancy whatever the results.

RHESUS NEGATIVE WOMEN

The Rhesus gene is attached to the red cells of the blood and is present in 85 per cent of the population. Rhesus negative women don't have this gene. This means that one in ten couples will consist of a Rhesus negative woman and a Rhesus positive man. This is fine if the baby is Rhesus negative, too, but if the baby is Rhesus positive there may be problems. At delivery if too much of the baby's blood gets into the mother's system, the mother creates special antibodies to destroy Rhesus positive cells. The next pregnancy can then be a problem if the baby is Rhesus positive again. As the baby develops the maternal antibodies increase and cross from the mother to the fetus and destroy its blood cells. The baby gets anaemic, jaundiced and swollen; untreated it will die.

This situation was very common until the invention of Anti D immunoglobulin (C,D, and E are all part of the Rhesus gene, D causes the problems). This mops up any stray Rhesus positive blood cells in the circulation before the mother starts producing her damaging antibodies. Anti D is given at birth, after a threatened miscarriage or any other bleeding.

Rhesus babies are now rare, but some women do develop antibodies without warning. If the baby becomes affected and anaemic, blood transfusions can be given directly into the baby's umbilical cord with guidance from an ultrasound scanning machine.

SICKLE-CELL DISEASE/THALASSEMIA

Sickle-cell disease is normally found in women with origins in the Middle East, Africa and the West Indies, and it can only be inherited when both parents carry the trait. *Thalassemia* is similar to sickle-cell disease, and affects people from Mediterranean countries, the Middle East, India and Pakistan. Sickle-cell disease means that the haemoglobin part of the red cell (the bit that carries the oxygen) is deformed. When the red blood cells become short of oxygen, for example when over-exercising or during an infection, they become sickle shaped, disrupting circulation, and causing severe pain. It can be diagnosed in the fetus by chorionic villus sampling (CVS, see below).

Pregnancy can cause more complications in women with sickle-cell disease, with increased risk of high blood pressure and infection problems. The abnormal haemoglobin can also affect the placenta, resulting in a small and poorly nourished baby. Close ante-natal care is essential for women with sickle-cell disease.

DOWN'S SYNDROME

Down's syndrome happens when there is an extra chromosome 21 (there are normally 46 chromosomes in a fertilised egg, a Down's baby has 47). Children born with Down's syndrome have some degree of mental handicap, and often other abnormalities as well. They have slanting eyes which accounts for the original name, mongolism.

If you're under thirty the risk of having a Down's syndrome baby is less than one in a 1000. This risk increases with age, to more than one in fifty if you're over forty-five. The age of the mother seems more important than the age of the father, although this may also be a contributing factor. Most units offer screening tests to women aged thirty-five or over, not because the risk dramatically goes up then (it's one in 350), but because there has to be a sensible cut-off point. If you're under thirty-five and really worried about having a Down's baby, talk to your consultant – most are sympathetic.

CHORIONIC VILLUS SAMPLING (CVS) CVS is a relatively recent method for diagnosing Down's syndrome, which is done when you're about nine weeks pregnant. There are two methods: through the vagina by passing a fine tube up through the cervix into the uterus, or through the abdomen with a fine needle directly into the uterus. With the help of a scanning machine to check position, the needle or tube sucks up a very small bit of placenta (chorionic villus). There may be a little discomfort but it's soon over. The result is available in a matter of days.

The miscarriage rate is between 2 and 4 per cent but this value may be high because before twelve weeks your chances of miscarrying are higher anyway. There's been a recent report of fetal damage after doing CVS through the abdomen, so the results of a large trial going on are awaited anxiously.

The great advantage of this technique is that if you opt for a termination after the result it can be done by the suction technique (page 96) quickly and easily.

AMNIOCENTESIS This method is used to diagnose a range of disorders including Down's syndrome. It's usually done at sixteen weeks and involves passing a fine needle through the abdomen (which may first be frozen with local anaesthetic) to a puddle of amniotic fluid visible on the scan. Some women feel quite scared exposing their abdomen to a long needle, but having had three of them myself I can say it's not bad at all. The fluid is sent off to the laboratory where the chromosomes are grown. This all takes time and means the result isn't available for three to four weeks. This means therefore that any decision to have a termination is made when you are almost twenty weeks pregnant and has to be by the induced labour method (page 97). The miscarriage rate is low, between 0.5 and 1 per cent.

AMNIOCENTESIS

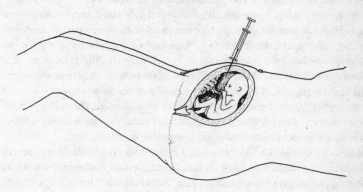

What's new
As most women over thirty-five are tested, the majority of babies born with Down's syndrome are of mothers under thirty-five. A new blood

test – *the triple test* – looks promising as a method of screening those women at risk. It measures three chemicals in the blood (including the alpha-fetaprotein which is raised in spina bifida), compares the results with the mother's age and length of pregnancy and works out the risk of a Down's baby. If the risk is high (about one in 150), an amniocentesis may be advised. The blood test can only suggest that there may be a problem – an amniocentesis will confirm this one way or the other. The test is done at sixteen weeks, so it would mean a late termination (page 97) if the chromosomes are abnormal. This may soon become available as a screening test for all women.

SPINA BIFIDA

Spina bifida is a defect in the development of the spine which leaves the spinal cord carrying precious nervous tissue exposed. If this happens in the skull the brain isn't covered, and the baby can't live for more than a few days. A defect lower down the spine can leave the baby paralysed and incontinent. Surgery after birth can help sometimes.

In this country four babies in every 1000 have some kind of spina bifida, more in Wales and Northern Ireland, less in the south of England. Diet and lack of vitamins are thought to be related to developing a spina bifida baby.

ALPHA-FETOPROTEIN TESTS Screening is done in some units with a blood test at sixteen weeks. The exposed nervous tissue leaks *alpha-fetoprotein* and gives a high result in the mother's blood. An amniocentesis is then necessary to see if the protein is high in the amniotic fluid. At the same time a scan is done to look carefully at the baby's spine. If these prove positive a termination is offered. (In some parts of the country an ultrasound scan alone is relied on to look closely at the spine and brain structure. This is done at eighteen to twenty weeks.)

If you've already had a spina bifida pregnancy you're ten times as likely to have another one. It's a good idea to take extra vitamins before you conceive next time. Recent research has shown folic acid taken before conception significantly reduces the chances of having a spina bifida baby if you've had one before. It's a vitamin naturally found in liver, kidneys, green vegetables, yeast, nuts and fruit.

THE ULTRASOUND SCAN

In the last ten years *ultrasound scanning* has become more and more sophisticated. Now you can tell which sex the baby is, watch it sucking it's thumb, and see clearly the development of its face.

ULTRASOUND SCAN

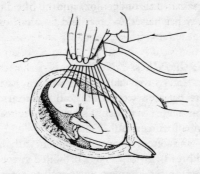

Many scan departments will arrange a routine scan at somewhere between eighteen and twenty weeks. The baby's head will be measured and this will be checked with your dates to see if your expected date of delivery is right. The spine will be carefully followed from the baby's head to its bottom. The heart will be checked for any abnormalities; the kidneys and bladder can also be seen. The thigh bones are measured and the other limbs checked.

Scan departments are usually very friendly places and often you can bring your partner along to watch with you. It's a fascinating experience. Scanning pregnancies has been done for twenty years now and seems entirely safe, but more research needs to be done on the possible long-term effects of ultrasound on the growing fetus.

THE FIRST TRIMESTER (FIRST 12 WEEKS)

Pregnancy is divided into three sections of roughly three months (trimesters), the first twelve weeks, twelve to twenty-eight weeks, and twenty-eight to forty weeks. The main organ development takes place in the first twelve weeks, the remainder of the time being spent growing and maturing.

At six weeks, the baby will have a head, brain and heart. The heart can sometimes be seen beating on a scan at this stage. Your period is only two weeks late. At eight weeks, the arms and legs are developing and beginning to move; the

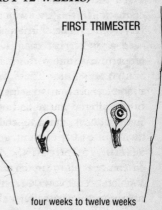

FIRST TRIMESTER

four weeks to twelve weeks

face has formed with eyes and ears. At twelve weeks the baby now weighs about 30 grams (just under 2oz) and all the internal organs are formed. The baby has hands and feet and usually lies curled up in a ball.

EARLY FEELINGS OF PREGNANCY

NAUSEA AND SICKNESS Over half of all women have nausea and vomiting somewhere between weeks four and fourteen of pregnancy. For some women this can be very depressing – you're really pleased to be pregnant, but you feel so awful. Don't go for long on an empty stomach, eat little and often, concentrating on carbohydrate meals (potatoes, pasta and bread). Barley sugars or boiled sweets can help the nausea between meals. In the morning don't rush to get up, try to have a few plain biscuits and a cup of tea first. Keep out of the kitchen and avoid major cooking if you can help it.

If you can't keep fluids down you may have to be admitted to hospital. You and the baby can survive quite well without food for some time, but without fluid you will become seriously dehydrated.

BLADDER TROUBLE Wanting to urinate frequently can be another sign of early pregnancy. You may have to get up in the night as well. This usually improves only to return in the later months as the baby's head pushes on to the bladder. Some women notice incontinence for the first time during pregnancy: it may happen as a combination of a full bladder and suddenly sneezing or coughing. This can be very embarrassing if away from home. Avoid letting your bladder get too full and remember to practise your pelvic floor exercises (page 150).

YOUR BREASTS In your first pregnancy the breast changes can be quite dramatic. In the first two or three months the breasts grow and can be very tender. The skin around the nipple may become darker. If you need a bigger bra even at this stage, make sure you are measured properly at a store with a maternity department.

STRETCH MARKS These are reddish lines that may appear on the abdomen, breasts and sometimes thighs and seem to be related as much to the altered hormone levels of pregnancy as to the growing baby. Some women expecting twins have none at all, other women develop them quite early on in pregnancy. Though various creams are marketed especially to prevent them no evidence has shown they make any difference at all to stretch marks.

VAGINAL DISCHARGE AND BLEEDING There is an increased blood supply to the vagina which makes it produce more secretions. Thrush (page 86) is more common in pregnancy: go to the doctor if the discharge is irritating, smelly or very heavy.

Spotting is common early in pregnancy, too, especially when the fertilised egg implants in the uterus at about the time your missed period is due. Some women think this is a normal but light period and don't realise they're pregnant. If you know you are pregnant any bleeding should be reported to your doctor or midwife.

CONSTIPATION Pregnancy hormones have a relaxing effect on the muscle wall of the bowel, which means that everything slows down. Iron tablets can make this worse. Make sure you have enough vegetables, fruit and fibre in your diet and plenty of fluids. If you have to take iron change to another preparation if it upsets your bowels.

BACKACHE More usually a feature of late pregnancy, backache at this stage may be a warning to take extra care. Sleep on a firm bed, wear flat heels, and be very careful about lifting shopping or the children. Again, the progesterone hormone is relaxing the supporting ligaments, making your back more vulnerable.

TEETH AND GUMS Hormones affect the make-up of the gum tissue, making them more prone to infection. The gums bleed more easily and can affect your teeth. Dental treatment is free, so make use of it if you're worried. Have a check-up anyway.

VARICOSE VEINS These can appear for the first time during pregnancy. The veins in your legs become swollen, lumpy and blue and can ache at the end of the day; it's best not to stand or sit still for long periods. Support tights may give relief, and you can get these on prescription.

PILES These are varicose veins around the anus and, again, may appear for the first time. They can bleed after having your bowels open and make your bottom itchy and sore. Your doctor can give you some soothing cream, but most important is to eat a high fibre diet (page 11) with plenty of fluids to make the motions soft and bulky.

EARLY PROBLEMS

BLEEDING AND MISCARRIAGE

Perhaps as many as one in three conceptions ends in miscarriage, which means it is much commoner than people think. A lot of these appear as a heavy period a little late and pregnancy isn't considered; 15 per cent of women miscarry a confirmed pregnancy. For someone who has been trying for a baby and had a positive pregnancy test, a miscarriage can be devastating.

Why does it happen?

Most miscarriages take place in the first three months and are usually a problem with development of the fetus at an early stage. Chromosome abnormalities are probably very common, and miscarrying is nature's way of dealing with the problem.

Sometimes the pregnancy appears as foreign to the mother's circulation and is rejected. Normally this reaction is blocked by the mother's antibodies. If the mother and father have more tissue characteristics in common than usual, the antibodies may not be produced and the pregnancy will miscarry.

Miscarriage can also occur if there are structural problems of the uterus and cervix. You wouldn't know about this necessarily without hospital tests (laparoscopy, page 47, or a hysterosalpingogram X-ray).

How do you miscarry?

Bleeding is usually the first sign followed by period-like pain. General advice is to rest and take things easy, although there isn't any scientific evidence that this prevents miscarriage. It's a good idea to stop sexual intercourse, too.

If the bleeding or pain becomes severe your doctor may send you into hospital or to the next available clinic. An ultrasound scan is essential to find out whether this is a good pregnancy or not. After six weeks the pregnancy is usually visible and a fetal heart beat can be seen. This is a very good sign and the chances of miscarrying fall dramatically.

If the bleeding and pain get worse this usually means the cervix is opening, allowing the pregnancy to pass through. This may look like pale, firm material, quite different from a blood clot. Sometimes the fetus is passed.

Some women miscarry at home. If this is the case, it's best to go into hospital for a check that everything has come away. This may involve a visit to the operating theatre or a scan. You normally need a D & C (page 50) to make sure all the tissue has gone. If this isn't done, the risks of infection and bleeding increase. The bleeding settles down after a week or so and a normal period arrives four to six weeks later.

The medical term for a miscarriage is a *spontaneous abortion*. The word abortion can be emotive, especially when you've lost a pregnancy, so don't be upset if you hear this mentioned by your doctor or when you are at the hospital. The other medical terms covering abortion are:

Threatened abortion – vaginal bleeding and pain
Incomplete abortion – only part of the pregnancy has been passed.
Complete abortion – all of the pregnancy has miscarried (uncommon)
Missed abortion – the fetus has died with no signs of miscarrying. An evacuation is necessary so that the body can get back to normal.
Recurrent abortion – this is where there have been three miscarriages in a row and can be very distressing. Reasons like those mentioned above are checked. Recent research has suggested that women who have high levels of the pituitary hormone LH (*luteinising hormone*) before conception takes place – in the first half of the cycle – may have an increased chance of miscarriage. Drugs that lower LH may prove very useful.

After any miscarriage the standard advice has been to leave things for three months before trying again, but it doesn't really matter. Just make sure you're fit and well and in the best possible shape for starting again. Coming to terms with losing a pregnancy is all part of this. You may feel guilty, sad, angry and even fearful; and you will certainly need the support of your partner, friends and family doctor.

For most women the chances of getting pregnant again are the same as before they miscarried, as are the chances of staying pregnant and giving birth to a normal baby.

> *If it hadn't been for my doctor's attitude I wouldn't have tried – every time I had a miscarriage he was as upset and concerned as me. After the third miscarriage he sent me to a specialist although he did stress that he wasn't concerned about my health – 50 per cent of conceptions are unsuccessful anyway, it's unfortunate but not dangerous, and not my body's fault.*
>
> *The consultant said there was nothing medically wrong with me. In a way that was worse – because it meant there was nothing I could do – it was out of my control.*
>
> *If my husband hadn't been so supportive I may not have got through it. Although I consider myself a fairly logical and detached person I wasn't because it was MY body.*
>
> *After the second loss I went for a scan – just to check I didn't need a D&C. When I went in the nurse asked me how many weeks pregnant I was – I felt very vulnerable. She hadn't been briefed properly or was having a bad day – but I felt that the people I was relying on were unemotionally involved – they see it all day. It would help if they were just a little more understanding.*
>
> *When I found out I was pregnant this time the midwife gave me*

*a number to contact the Miscarriage Association – I could have
done with that the first time around.*

Miscarriage Association, c/o Clayton Hospital, Northgate, Wakefield,
West Yorkshire WF1 3JS. Helpline Tel: 0924 200799.

ECTOPIC PREGNANCY

An *ectopic pregnancy* is a serious condition where the fertilised egg
implants in the Fallopian tube itself; it can also implant on the ovary or
even in the abdomen. As the embryo grows it gets too big for the tube,
which bursts with internal haemorrhage.

An ectopic pregnancy is more common if you have had a pelvic
infection in the past, take the progestogen-only Pill or have an IUD for
contraception. Older women seem more susceptible and if you've had
one ectopic pregnancy then the risks are much higher.

DIAGNOSIS It can be difficult to diagnose an ectopic pregnancy. There
is usually irregular bleeding following a missed period, abdominal
pain, perhaps just on one side, and doubtful pregnancy tests – negative
or weakly positive. An ultrasound scan may show an empty uterus and
possibly the ectopic pregnancy, but this is usually difficult to see.

TREATMENT Because of the risks of internal bleeding, if there's any
question of an ectopic pregnancy your doctor will want you to be in
hospital. A general and pelvic examination will be done and your blood
count checked. The pregnancy test and ultrasound scan should help
decide whether or not it's an ectopic pregnancy.

A laparoscopy (page 47) is done to confirm the diagnosis. Surgery is
required and the tube may have to be removed, although attempts are
made to save it if at all possible.

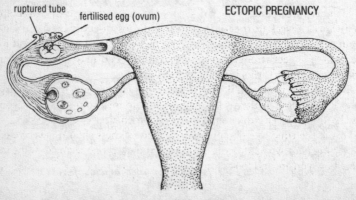

ruptured tube   fertilised egg (ovum)   ECTOPIC PREGNANCY

What's new

Recent techniques have been developed to avoid surgery and therefore cutting of the tube. A drug can be injected through the laparoscope which terminates the pregnancy. However, at present most gynaecologists remove the damaged part of the tube with surgery.

Afterwards it can be a difficult experience to get over: was it a real pregnancy, have I lost a baby, will it happen again? The grief reaction can be greater than that of a miscarriage and it's important to talk it through with your doctor.

Next time an early ultrasound scan will check that the pregnancy is in the uterus, so it's important to tell the doctor as soon as you think you're pregnant.

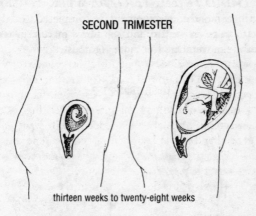

SECOND TRIMESTER

thirteen weeks to twenty-eight weeks

THE SECOND TRIMESTER (13th to 28th WEEK)

In the next three months the fetus grows in size and strength. At about the twentieth week (earlier with second and subsequent babies) you will begin to feel the baby kick: starting as a flutter, sometimes like wind in the bowel, it gets stronger and more definite. You may notice regular jerking movements; this is the baby hiccoughing.

Around this time you'll find it more difficult to get into ordinary jeans and skirts. The uterus is now growing up into your abdomen; you may be able to feel a ridge in the lower abdomen after twelve weeks.

This is the time to enjoy pregnancy. The sickness should have gone, you're pregnant without being enormous and everyone seems to want to know how you are and look after you.

MID-TERM PROBLEMS

PREMATURE LABOUR
Labour starting in the second trimester is definitely premature, although good Special Care baby units have had some successes with babies born as early as twenty-four weeks; for babies born at twenty-eight weeks and over the success rate increases. If you have any bleeding or regular contraction (tightening) pains, or if you feel a gush of water, you must get in touch with your midwife, doctor or maternity unit as soon as possible. Labour can be stopped if the pregnancy seems otherwise normal; a drip containing a uterus relaxing agent (ritodrine) may be necessary.

THE THIRD TRIMESTER (29th WEEK TO TERM)
In the last three months development is completed. In the last ten weeks the fetus puts on weight and the lungs mature in readiness for birth. The baby's movements feel more vigorous.

THIRD TRIMESTER

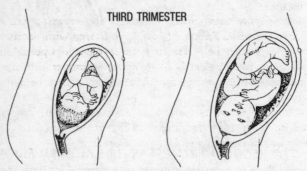

twenty-nine weeks to forty weeks

LATE COMPLAINTS

INDIGESTION AND HEARTBURN This can be quite a shock if you've never had indigestion before. It's caused by a combination of the relaxing effects of the pregnancy hormones on the stomach and the pressure exerted by the baby. Acid leaks up into the oesophagus and causes an unpleasant burning sensation.

Eat several small meals a day, avoid bending over, sleep propped up with pillows, and steer clear of rich, spicy foods. If it's still a problem your doctor will give you medicine to neutralise the acid and protect the oesophagus (Asilone, Gaviscon).

INCREASED SWEATING Your blood circulation will be super-dynamic late on in pregnancy. You won't feel the cold so much, but you may find that getting warm makes you perspire more than normal. You may find you get damp between the legs as well. This is absolutely normal. A cool shower and change of cotton clothes will make you feel more comfortable. Be careful in the bath: water that is too hot may make you feel faint, especially when you stand up.

SLEEPING DIFFICULTIES It's hardly surprising that it's difficult to get comfortable with a baby kicking inside you. Avoid a large meal last thing at night, stop drinking coffee and cola drinks altogether, and restrict your tea intake. Have a warm milk drink and relaxing warm bath before bed if you feel like it. Make sure the bed is firm and you have plenty of pillows. Sleep upright if heartburn is a problem. Lying on your back may make you feel faint and affect the baby's circulation in late pregnancy – it puts pressure on the major blood vessels. Sleeping on your side may be more comfortable if you have a pillow between your legs.

Cramp is more common in pregnancy: don't restrict your legs and feet with tucked-in sheets. Elevating your legs with another pillow under your feet may help. Having your feet and legs gently massaged can help, too. Restless legs is another sleep preventer, difficult to treat but paracetamol or a very mild sleeping tablet may help if you are desperate.

Lack of sleep can be very soul destroying, both mentally and physically. Talk to your doctor if it's a real problem, she may recommend mild sleeping tablets for a short time.

One in ten women feel quite out of breath in the last couple of months of pregnancy. Some get nosebleeds more frequently. Backache, varicose veins, bladder weakness and piles may all get more troublesome towards the end of pregnancy.

CHECKING THE BABY FOR GROWTH

At each visit to the clinic your abdomen and the size of the baby will be checked. You may be measured from the top of the pelvic bone to the top of the uterus with a tape measure.

ULTRASOUND SCAN Some clinics do a second ultrasound scan at around thirty to thirty-two weeks to make sure the baby is growing normally.

The head measurement is not so important now, but the baby's waist measurement is a good guide to its nourishment; so is the amount of amniotic fluid.

DOPPLER SCANS If there's any doubt about the baby's growth a *Doppler scan* may be arranged. This measures the flow in the blood vessels in the umbilical cord and in the baby itself. If the flow is reduced there may be a problem with growth.

CTG (CARDIOTOCOGRAPH) You will be asked in the clinic if the baby is moving normally. If the baby has been quiet, it's a good idea to monitor the heart beat with a CTG. This is usually done in hospital. The heart beat is recorded from an ultrasound disc on your abdomen and you note when the baby is moving. The resulting trace will indicate everything is all right.

The baby's movements are very important: don't ignore them. If you think the baby is quiet, sit down and relax for an hour or two. If the movements are still not right seek help from the midwife or hospital.

Small babies which are not growing properly can be quite a problem. Poor growth can be due to smoking, fetal infection or abnormality, high blood pressure in the mother or for no apparent reason. Adequate rest is important and the baby closely monitored with heart tracings, scans and Doppler measurements; you may need to stay in hospital for these. It will be a careful balance working out when the baby will be better off in the outside world, especially if there is a major problem before thirty-two weeks, as the baby is quite premature.

A recent study in France has looked at mothers who had had one growth-retarded baby in the past. Those given a low dose of aspirin in the next pregnancy had significantly bigger babies than those who took a dummy drug. Aspirin seems to prevent the hormonal changes that damage placental arteries in some women.

LATE-TERM PROBLEMS

PREGNANCY INDUCED HYPERTENSION (PIH)

At the clinic your blood pressure (BP) and urine will be checked. An increase in BP and the appearance of protein in the urine can mean you're developing *Pregnancy Induced Hypertension* (PIH). This used to be called *toxaemia* or *pre-eclampsia*. It's associated with swelling of the ankles and fingers, but this is very common in normal pregnancy.

If rest at home doesn't improve things you may have to go into hospital where BP lowering drugs may be given. Checks will also be done on the protein in your urine. With severe PIH the placenta works less well and the baby's growth may be affected. Delivery may be considered before your due date either by inducing labour or by doing a caesarean section.

Research has suggested that a low dose of ordinary aspirin taken every day from early in pregnancy will help to prevent PIH developing.

VAGINAL BLEEDING

This is always taken seriously in pregnancy. Much of the time the bleeding can't really be accounted for and quite frequently it's due to a minor problem with the cervix such as a polyp (page 57) or cervical erosion (page 31), or with the vagina (thrush, page 86). The two major problems are *placenta praevia* and *placental abruptio*.

Placenta praevia This can be a dangerous condition because the placenta lies low down in front of the baby's way out of the uterus. With more and more women having ultrasound scans which check the placenta, the days of severe and dramatic bleeding from a surprise placenta praevia are rare. If your placenta is low you may need a repeat scan in a few weeks to check; it can move out of the way as the uterus grows in late pregnancy. If it is still a problem you may have to go into hospital in case of bleeding, and delivery is by caesarean section at around thirty-eight weeks.

Placental abruptio This bleeding can be serious, endangering both mother and baby. For some unknown reason the placenta shears off from one edge, releasing blood; some leaks outside, some stays inside and causes pain. Because the baby's life-support system has been disrupted, there may be fetal distress or, if too late, a dead baby. In severe cases the treatment is to deliver the baby as soon as possible, encouraging labour or doing an emergency caesarean section.

A 'show' – consisting of jelly-like mucus streaked with blood – is not strictly bleeding. It's common at the onset of labour, after a vaginal examination in late pregnancy or when the baby's head is going down in the pelvis.

GETTING READY FOR LABOUR

In the last four weeks of pregnancy you'll be making preparations for the baby's arrival. Some women feel a great nesting instinct, painting and decorating, buying linen and furniture, sewing and knitting. Some find it very difficult to concentrate, are forgetful, and unable to follow the plot of a film or book. This is supposed to get you into the right mentality for caring for the very young as a top priority. It can be unnerving if you're still working, or coping, say, with the older children's difficult homework.

The mild tightenings, known as *Braxton-Hicks contractions*, that have been going on throughout pregnancy, get more noticeable in the last few weeks. Some of these can be quite uncomfortable. They don't necessarily mean labour is starting they may just be helping to push the baby's head down into the pelvis. Labour pains increase in strength and frequency and don't fade away.

Engagement of the baby's head can be felt when your abdomen is examined. If more than half the baby's head is felt, the head isn't engaged; if less than half is felt it is. You can tell if the baby's head is well down, as there is more pressure on your bladder making you urinate more frequently, and you may feel generally uncomfortable when walking any distance. The head being engaged is a good sign that the baby's fitting in well and can mean an easy labour, but not being engaged certainly doesn't mean things are going to be difficult. A 'show' is common in late pregnancy but doesn't necessarily mean labour is starting.

It is very reassuring to see where you will be giving birth (unless you're planning a home birth). Parentcraft classes may arrange a guided tour of the labour ward; if not, ask the hospital midwife when you could look round. You'll be given details of what you'll need to bring in for yourself and the baby; most women have a case packed ready in the last month.

BIRTH PLAN

HOME BIRTH

Most family doctors are unhappy about looking after women who are having a baby at home – there will always be the risk of things going wrong for the mother and the baby. If a baby is born and fails to breathe it may need skilled resuscitation, which is only available at the maternity hospital precious minutes away. Unfortunately, no one can reliably predict which baby will be like this. It's unlikely if you're fit and have had a straightforward pregnancy and normal labour already, but it can happen. So can sudden, very heavy vaginal bleeding after the baby is born; this can threaten the mother's life if not dealt with promptly. In these days of smaller families, couples and their doctors may not be prepared to take the risk.

All this can make it difficult for the women who are convinced that a home birth is right for them despite the risks. In Holland half of all babies are born at home with very few problems, but this is a different population from the United Kingdom with possibly better health care in general. Independent midwives practising outside the National Health Service offer support and help to women who want to be delivered at home.

Talk to your midwife, she may know what the options are in your locality. For a doctor to accept you for a home birth you must be at the lowest possible risk of anything going wrong. If you've proved you can have a trouble-free pregnancy, labour and delivery before, then you are more likely to get support for a home birth from your doctor than someone in her first pregnancy. If there is an emergency obstetric unit – flying squad – operating in your area, all the better.

> *I decided I wanted a home birth because I had a bad experience in hospital the first time round with my son. I told my GP I was pregnant, and that I was thinking of a home delivery – he was anxious for me because he didn't think I'd get the care I needed – he was conscious of the problems because his wife had had a home delivery and there had been problems – but he did say that he would never say no to anybody. He told me to talk to the midwife. She said it was too early to make a decision as I was only nine and a half weeks pregnant, and there might be complications.*
>
> *On every visit I said I still wanted a home delivery. I saw the midwife – she said she hadn't done a home delivery before but would. We built up quite a good relationship.*
>
> *Three months before the birth my doctor wrote to me saying that following discussions with his partners they had decided that they couldn't offer GP cover for home delivery. My midwife became pregnant, which meant a new one was to be appointed.*
>
> *I met the new midwife – the first consultation was not good – she was worried. I came home in tears. Two days later she visited me at home with an assistant. I had to confirm that I would go into hospital at any point if there were complications. She wanted me to sign a document saying this. She made me feel so anxious – I said 'all I want from you is encouragement and support to help me through this.'*

On returning to the surgery it became obvious that she was not keen for a home delivery at all. She just kept making notes on my birth card records. I came out of the consultation in tears – I didn't trust her, and she wasn't interested at all. I couldn't have faced a delivery with that midwife, or in hospital. I felt so desperate, with only a few weeks of pregnancy I didn't know what to do.

I rang all over the country, I spoke to seven people. I eventually spoke to The Association of Radical Midwives. They gave me a contact in Bristol, the only independent midwife in the area. I called her in the evening, and told her my story. She said I was a classic case, a pregnant woman only given negative reaction on the subject of home birth. She wasn't sure if she could take me on at first. She rang the next morning; asked a few more questions. Asked me to visit her that evening with my husband, after all we both had to work together. She agreed to work for us.

She taught us both birth positions around my home, breathing. She spent one morning trying to get to know me. She didn't carry pethidine or any drugs. I was in labour for twenty hours. I trusted her with my life – and my baby's. My husband felt relaxed with her. She relaxed us all. I did the breathing she taught me, when I lost my way she would patiently remind me again. She didn't keep examining me – she said we should get into the 'birth atmosphere'. If I got uptight she would massage me – not offer me drugs.

She treated me wonderfully, gave me the confidence I wanted. She examined me eventually – I had dilated 6cm which I got to on my own! She told me I would cope – even when I was having a problem – she was firm and supportive – took me through the difficult, painful patches. I had no stitches and a drug free delivery. It was a normal, physiological birth.

NATURAL BIRTH

Two French obstetricians have pioneered alternative ways of giving birth, Frederick Leboyer and Michel Odent. Both have advocated ways of childbirth where the arrival of the baby is done with the minimum of trauma, into a warm, quiet, softly lit room. This may make it a very pleasant experience for all involved, but there hasn't been any proven benefit to mother and baby over a conventional birth. Their work, however, did make conventional obstetricians and midwives question the need for all the technical equipment and bright lights and noise that goes with a hospital delivery.

Odent maintains women have a natural nesting instinct to find a dark corner to deliver their babies. He stresses the importance of finding comfortable positions in labour; he prefers the supported squat for delivery, mother's knees apart and bent, supported under the arms by her partner or midwife.

Leboyer has advocated water births, which continue the principle of making the birth process more gradual and gentle. The mother relaxes in warm water through her labour and with the help of a midwife delivers the baby into the water (usually in the kneeling position holding on to the side of the bath). The baby is then taken up and into the mother's arms. The warm water certainly has a soothing effect on the contractions, but if the mother needs any other pain relief the water birth idea has to be abandoned. This would also be the case if there is any problem with the baby.

There seems no advantage in keeping the baby under water: it may get cold, or may try to gasp and inhale the water. The mother gets out of the bath to deliver the placenta.

If this appeals to you talk to the hospital midwife about it and see if it's possible in your unit. Most maternity units haven't a suitable bath installed, but it is possible to hire one to be kept until delivery (the hospital should have all the details).

Anxiety produces *catecholamines* – *adrenaline* and *noradrenaline* – which are the chemicals of the fight or flight response. These have a labour-suppressing effect on the uterus; if you're worried and uptight things may not go smoothly. If you have confidence in yourself and the people looking after you, there's a greater chance of a perfectly normal labour. It's best to be open and cope with whatever comes your way. If you're all set for a natural labour – read all the books, brought in the beanbag and soft music – and then the baby is distressed, try to accept that that's how it is, even if it means a caesarean section.

Active Birth Movement, 18 Laurier Road, London NW5 1SN. Tel: 071-267 3006. Details about pool hire and natural birth teachers.
National Childbirth Trust, Alexandra House, Oldham Terrace, Acton, London W3 6NH. Tel: 081-992 8637. Information about natural childbirth and lists of local groups.

HOSPITAL BIRTH
Over 95 per cent of births take place in hospital and a welcome result of this has been that many hospitals have made a real effort to be

welcoming and homely, questioning the need for many things done as routine in the past (such as shaving and enemas). The best way of finding out what's going on in your unit is to go to the ante-natal classes, look around the place and ask questions.

Some prospective mothers feel better writing down what they would like as a birth plan. Many clinics will provide you with a form to fill in, or you can just write down what you would like in labour.

– Mention what is worrying you. Say if you want your partner with you as much as possible – most labour wards expect this these days, it's the exceptions that sit it out in the corridor.

– If you feel strongly about your waters being broken in labour say so. It's standard practice in many places and can help your progress, but it can also increase the strength and frequency of the contractions.

– Say what you feel like for pain relief.

– Do you want to walk around in labour, do you want to deliver on the bed, or have a go at squatting or standing up?

– Do you feel strongly about monitoring the fetal heart – some places have the monitor running all the time, others just listen in with a trumpet at regular intervals. It doesn't seem to make a difference to the wellbeing of the baby.

– The episiotomy debate is quieter these days – this is the cut made in the perineum to enable the head to be born safely. Midwives do their utmost to avoid an unnecessary cut, but it means that tears do occasionally happen. You have to trust the midwife on the day to do what's best for you.

– Feeding. Mention if you would like the baby to go to the breast straight after birth. Do you want the baby only to have breast milk? Some units tend to offer bottles at night if the baby is unsettled.

Take the plan to the clinic and check it over with the doctor and midwife. It will go in your notes ready for when you arrive in labour.

GIVING BIRTH

Working out when you're actually in labour may not be as easy as it sounds. Doctors reckon that when you're having regular painful contractions which open the cervix then that's labour. A contraction is a tightening of the uterus which can be painful and can be felt by putting a hand on the abdomen. Contractions start off as a period pain, build up to a peak and then fade away over a spell of 60 to 90 seconds. Quite often strong contractions are simply practice ones and don't achieve anything as far as the cervix is concerned. These contractions can cause a 'show' (page 123). Again, this doesn't necessarily mean labour has really started. Sometimes labour begins with only the waters breaking. If contractions don't follow within a day, they are stimulated with an oxytocin drip or prostaglandin pessary. This is to prevent infection travelling from the vagina to the baby.

GOING TO HOSPITAL

When you go into hospital a midwife will be allocated to look after you. She will ask you what's happening and make her own assessment. She will need to take your temperature, pulse and blood pressure. Then the midwife will see how the contractions are behaving; as she is talking to you she will be noting how frequently they're coming and how you're reacting to the pain.

If the midwife is convinced you're in labour she may well go on to examine you internally; this can also check if your waters have broken. A vaginal examination in labour can be quite sore so the midwife will

FETAL POSITIONS IN LATE PREGNANCY

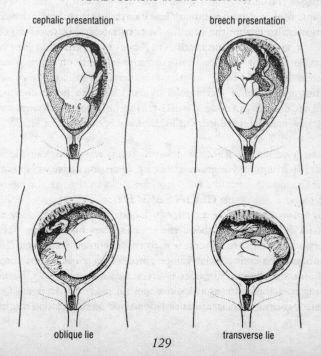

cephalic presentation

breech presentation

oblique lie

transverse lie

be as gentle as possible. She will feel for the cervix to see if it's dilating (opening) and for the baby's head to check how far down in the pelvis it has moved.

If you've not had your bowels open for a few days or the midwife feels motions in the rectum (easy to feel through the back wall of the vagina) she may recommend you have suppositories or a small enema. This means you've emptied the rectum by the time the baby is being born, otherwise it's delivered alongside faeces. Shaving the pubic hair has been abandoned these days.

Once in labour the stomach stops functioning normally and it's not safe to eat (vomiting solid food can be very dangerous in labour). You will be given sips of water or ice to suck.

FIRST STAGE OF LABOUR

If you're having true labour contractions the cervix will dilate from being closed or nearly closed to opening up completely (ultimately to 10 cm/4 in wide). Normally if you're in labour and the cervix is more than 4 cm/1½ in dilated the midwife will consider breaking your waters. This doesn't hurt; there are no nerves in the amniotic membranes. However, you should make it clear beforehand if you do not want your waters broken artificially; this is standard practice in some hospitals. If the amniotic fluid contains *meconium* (staining from the baby's bowel) extra care is taken to look for fetal distress in the baby from its heart rate.

The first stage of labour lasts until the cervix is fully dilated and the midwife can't feel any cervix at all, just the baby's head. Getting to 5 cm/2 in dilated can take a while (anything from 3–8 hours), after that things usually speed up, with the cervix opening at an ideal rate of 1 cm/½ in an hour.

If you need anything for the pain discuss it with your midwife; she may feel that you're doing so well and progressing so quickly that gas and air (Entonox) would be enough. If it looks as though the labour is going to be a long time perhaps pethidine (page 134) or an epidural (page 134) would be a better choice.

In the first stage of labour try to conserve your energy for the delivery. Try relaxing, shoulders down and arms and legs heavy, throughout each contraction. Concentrate on deep and regular breathing: count up to ten and back, recite a favourite song in your head, anything to get you through this contraction ready for the next one. At this stage, contractions last between 40 and 90 seconds, occurring every

CHILDBIRTH

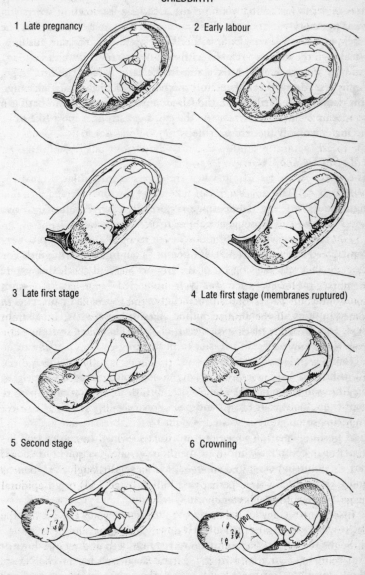

1 Late pregnancy   2 Early labour

3 Late first stage   4 Late first stage (membranes ruptured)

5 Second stage   6 Crowning

7 Birth of the head   8 Birth of the shoulders

3–5 minutes. As the cervix gets near to full dilation you may feel a strange sensation filling your pelvis, a bit like the feeling when you want to empty your bowels. This pushing feeling may come before the cervix is ready; your midwife will tell you when you can start pushing. Until then try and keep relaxed with each contraction, it won't be long.

Many women like to walk about in the early part of the first stage; doing something helps them to cope with the contractions, although this doesn't necessarily make the labour any quicker. A warm bath can be soothing for some women. As the pains get stronger most like to be sitting down or lying on their side.

THE SECOND STAGE

The second stage lasts from when the cervix is fully dilated until the baby is born. The first stage can take quite a while (average duration eight hours) but the second stage is normally over within one to two hours. Second and subsequent babies are usually quicker.

You usually have a tremendous desire to push as though you were constipated when the second stage begins. Your midwife will guide you through this very exciting bit of the labour. She will check that you're ready to push and then get you organised in a position most comfortable for you. Discuss this earlier on. If you've had pain relief in the form of an injection of pethidine or an epidural your legs may be weak and the safest place to deliver is on the bed, sitting upright or on your side. You may find it easier to push while you're squatting or on all fours, see what your midwife says.

Pushing is hard work. As a contraction starts prepare yourself by breathing in and out. Then take a deep breath in, drop your chin on to your chest, hold your breath and push down steadily. It's best to close your lips so no effort is wasted. Count to ten, breathe out and in and start pushing again. You won't want to push when the contraction has gone; relax completely and wait for the next one. Contractions should now be occurring every 2–3 minutes, and generally last for between 60 and 90 seconds.

Getting the hang of pushing can take a while, and your midwife may get you a mirror so you can see up the vagina and watch the baby's head move when you're pushing correctly.

When the baby is very nearly born the head will be very low down at the vaginal entrance (crowning). At this stage you have to be careful about pushing: too much will propel the baby's head out and risk tearing the perineum (the skin between the vagina and the anus) badly.

It usually takes a combination of small pushes and a lot of panting (quick shallow breaths) for the baby to be delivered. The midwife will be controlling the baby's head throughout.

If the perineum, which is very stretchy skin, looks as though it's beginning to tear the midwife may inject some local anaesthetic and make a small cut from the back of the vagina to one side, usually to the right (*episiotomy*). The baby's head is then eased out – you may be able to see this – and the body follows rapidly. The baby will still be attached to you by the umbilical cord, which the midwife cuts (this is a painless procedure), and then the baby is yours. If the baby is having difficulty starting breathing, it may need oxygen from a nearby resuscitating machine. This is important as lack of oxygen can cause brain damage.

THE THIRD STAGE

The third stage lasts from when the baby is born until the placenta is delivered. Many units give an injection (Syntometrine) to help the placenta come away quickly with the minimum of blood loss. This is given into your thigh just as the baby's body is being born.

After delivery the midwife will gently pull on the umbilical cord and deliver the placenta. This looks like a large piece of liver and will be checked to make sure it's all there; any left behind in the uterus may cause bleeding and infection.

You'll be exhausted, exhilarated and amazed. If you feel like it you can see if the baby wants to suckle at the breast. You won't be producing milk yet but a yellowish fluid called colostrum. This may have been leaking from the nipples in the last half of pregnancy. It's high in antibodies so probably helps the baby cope against infection in the early days. Suckling will also help the uterus contract, separate the placenta if it's still attached, and help the uterus to return to its normal size.

The area where the placenta was attached is left raw and this bleeds for a few weeks, gradually decreasing in amount. Heavy bleeding and pain in the days and weeks after delivery may suggest there is infection. This is often caused by a little piece of placenta left behind. Treatment involves antibiotics and a return to hospital for the uterus to be checked and cleaned as with a D & C (page 50).

PAIN RELIEF

Breathing and relaxation classes will teach you simple methods of coping with the pain. But labour can be long and most women having their first baby find they need help with the stronger contractions.

GAS AND AIR (ENTONOX) This is inhaled by the mother herself using a face mask when the contraction is coming and as long as it lasts. As it contains 50 per cent nitrous oxide and 50 per cent oxygen it's probably beneficial for the baby and is great for coping with the climax of a short sharp labour.

PETHIDINE An analgesic, which is given by injection and makes you feel drowsy, taking the edge off the pain. It lasts for two to three hours. It does get through to the baby, also making it drowsy, and can affect the heart rate tracing. There aren't any serious long-term consequences of this and pethidine has been used in labour for many years. If the baby is born with pethidine still in its system and is reluctant to breathe, an injection is given which reverses its effect (Naloxone).

EPIDURAL Ideal for long labours or when labour is induced, an epidural anaesthesia can take the pain away completely. An injection in the back sends local anaesthetic to the nerves going to the abdomen and legs, so you feel numb from the waist down with heavy legs. A fine tube is left in place and further anaesthetic is given when the pains come back. Pushing can be more difficult if you don't have the strong urge to push; the midwife will tailor the dose to help you with this. If you need a forceps delivery or your baby is breech (bottom first) then this is the most comfortable pain relief available.

EPIDURAL

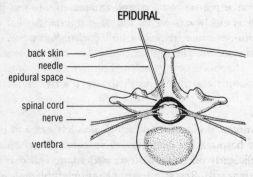

back skin
needle
epidural space
spinal cord
nerve
vertebra

A small amount of this local anaesthetic does get through to the baby, but it doesn't seem to cause any problems. The changes in your blood circulation with an epidural can drop your blood pressure dramatically sometimes; the baby won't like this and may react by dropping its heart rate. This can easily be solved by increasing the fluid coming to you in a drip (essential if you want an epidural).

A large study of women who'd had epidurals showed an increase in back problems afterwards. This was thought to be due to the positioning of the legs during labour. When you have an epidural your legs can be quite numb so you have no control of where they are and what is comfortable. If the legs are not properly supported, as you would do if you could feel them, it may place a strain on the back. It's a good idea therefore to have a pillow between your legs when you're lying on your side.

TRANSCUTANEOUS ELECTRICAL NERVE STIMULATOR (*TENS*) This is only available in some units (contact your local NCT group). Electrode pads are placed on the lower back and a mild electric current switched on during a contraction. This causes a gentle tingling sensation and if the current is increased gives some pain relief. It definitely helps some women, but if the labour is difficult or prolonged then usually extra pain relief is necessary.

ALTERNATIVE METHODS Hypnosis and acupuncture are well known and effective forms of pain relief in the East. Availability depends on your locality, ask your midwife if she knows anyone prepared to be involved in your labour pain relief. There would be a charge for this.

Every woman is different in the way she copes with pain. It's much better if you're confident and relaxed; the effect of pain is certainly worsened by fear. Approach labour with an open mind. You may want a natural birth as much as possible, but if on the day it's not meant to be don't feel guilty or that it's your fault. The main thing is that both you and the baby are well, fit and healthy.

LABOUR AND DELIVERY COMPLICATIONS

INDUCTION

The most common reason for inducing labour is that the baby is overdue. Most hospitals are concerned that the placenta will not feed the baby so efficiently once you are two weeks late, and that therefore the pregnancy is at risk. Research has not confirmed this, however.

Some women welcome induced labour when the days start to drag on and they are desperate to get things started. If you feel you want to go into labour naturally, even though you are overdue, discuss it with your consultant: most would be sympathetic if the baby was healthy inside.

If you have other problems, like high blood pressure or poor fetal growth, an induction may be suggested as the best course of action.

ARTIFICIAL RUPTURE OF MEMBRANES (ARM) A vaginal examination is done to assess the state of the cervix. If it's 2 – 3 cm/¾ – 1¼ in open, and the doctor can feel the baby's head through it, it may be easy to get you into labour by breaking your waters (*artificial rupture of the amniotic membranes*). This is done as part of an internal examination with a plastic hook – it doesn't hurt as there is no sensation in the amniotic membranes. Having done this, contractions may start on their own if you were almost going into labour anyway.

OXYTOCIN If the contractions still don't start, you will need a drip containing oxytocin (Syntocinon) – an artificial hormone like the one you produce in a natural labour.

PROSTAGLANDIN PESSARIES If the cervix is long and closed or not easily accessible by the examining finger, the induction is started with a prostaglandin pessary (Prostin) or some gel. Natural prostaglandins help to start off normal labour, so these preparations can mimic a fairly normal start to labour. They will either open up the cervix sufficiently for the waters to be broken or actually put you into labour. The baby will be monitored with a fetal heart monitor intermittently.

An induced labour, especially if it's your first baby, can be quite long. If you find the pains difficult to cope with early on, the most comfortable pain relief would be an epidural (page 134).

DISADVANTAGES Some mothers (2 per cent) just won't go into labour. If either the mother or baby is at risk by continuing the pregnancy a caesarean section must be done.

Induced labours are said to be longer, need more pain relief, and end up with a higher risk of caesarean section or forceps delivery. This is much less common now with the widespread use of prostaglandins.

FORCEPS DELIVERY

There used to be a rule about the second stage: no longer than an hour. Midwives are more relaxed about this these days and if you're getting there and the baby's head is coming down then no one is going to watch the clock.

But pushing, after maybe a very tiring first stage and perhaps sleepless nights before going into labour, is exhausting if it goes on for long. It may also mean there are problems. The baby's head may be turned to the side (*transverse position*) and this way is too big to deliver. Normally, the baby is looking at the floor when you're lying down. The baby must be turned to look down before it's delivered.

Depending on how the baby's heart rate is behaving, there may be

FORCEPS DELIVERY

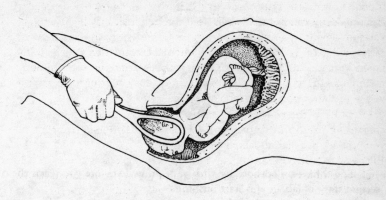

time to get you quite comfortable with an epidural (page 134) or spinal anaesthetic (injection directly into the spinal cord), so you don't feel any discomfort. If time is limited the doctor will give you an injection of local anaesthetic into the nerves at the top of the vagina.

Your legs will have to be bent up and wide apart, with your feet supported in stirrups. Metal forceps or a vacuum cap (Ventouse) are then put on the baby's head, turning it if necessary, and the baby delivered with your help, pushing with contractions. The baby's body is then delivered normally. An episiotomy is almost always done.

The baby may have small marks on its head from the forceps, or a swelling in the scalp from the vacuum, but these are nothing to worry about, and will settle down after a few days.

EPISIOTOMY

An *episiotomy* is a cut made with scissors at an angle from the back of the vaginal entrance in the area called the perineum (the area is injected with local anaesthetic first so it doesn't hurt). It enables the head of the baby to be born more easily and quickly and avoids tearing. It's necessary if you have a forceps delivery because of the extra space taken up by the forceps blades.

There has been some recent debate about episiotomies and the need for them. It was thought they were being done too frequently, with no warning, and for no good reason. In fact, most midwives and doctors take the view that if it is possible to get away without an episiotomy, even if it leaves a small tear, then so much the better. Discuss whether

EPISIOTOMY

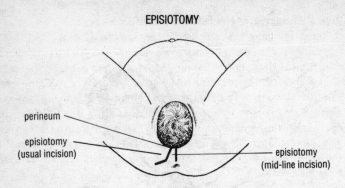

perineum

episiotomy
(usual incision)

episiotomy
(mid-line incision)

you should have an episiotomy with your midwife before you reach the second stage of labour and start pushing.

The healing process and the stitches used to repair the cut do cause some discomfort afterwards – it may be difficult to walk normally and sit straight in the first few days. An episiotomy takes about two to three weeks to heal, and intercourse may be quite sore at the first attempt. Some women have trouble with intercourse for some time after. A new method of repairing episiotomies, using an adhesive glue (Histoacryl) for the outside layer (so no external stitches), has been tried in Israel and looks promising. Certain kinds of catgut (glycerol impregnated catgut) seem to cause a lot more problems than other suture material. An invisible, under-the-skin stitch is much more comfortable than individual external stitches.

CAESAREAN SECTION

Everyone hopes the delivery of her baby will go as smoothly and normally as possible, but there is always the chance if things don't go to plan that a *caesarean section* may be necessary.

Despite the recent popular interest in natural childbirth, the caesarean section rate has gone up and up. From being one in twenty-two deliveries in 1962, it jumped to one in nine in 1985 and is still increasing. We seem to be catching the USA up all the time (it's one in five there). Unfortunately, the fear of being sued has affected obstetricians' practice. It is sometimes simpler to do a caesarean section than risk a difficult forceps delivery and suffer litigation. However, recent evidence has shown that many brain-damaged babies are damaged before birth and not because of the birth process. This may temper the soaring caesarean rate.

When a caesarean is necessary

Sometimes the baby gets stuck, the cervix stops dilating, and there is no progress. An oxytocin (Syntocinon) drip (page 136) can improve the contractions if they are not strong enough, and an epidural (page 134) can relax and rest the mother. If, however, the cervix still won't fully dilate then the only way to deliver the baby is by caesarean. The main reason for this is that the head of the baby is too big for the pelvis; sometimes this is because it's lying in an awkward position. As making the decision to do a caesarean takes some time, it's sometimes possible to have the section done under an epidural and be awake with your partner beside you.

CAESAREAN SECTION

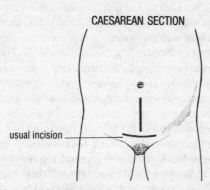

usual incision

The other major reason for doing a caesarean section is because the baby is distressed. If the fetal heart tracing, which is checked throughout labour, occasionally shows decreases in the heart rate, this could mean distress. Sometimes the baby's blood chemistry is checked first, sometimes it's safer to do a caesarean section as quickly as possible. This means a general anaesthetic.

The caesarean section

The operation takes about forty minutes in total, but the baby is born within ten minutes. The incision is made in the bikini line and heals very well; it's surprisingly comfortable compared to an episiotomy (having had both myself).

You'll be on your feet the next day trying a gentle walk and usually home after a week or so. The wound takes at least six weeks to heal internally, so avoid heavy lifting (young children included).

Having one caesarean doesn't always mean you have to have another section; discuss it with your obstetrician. However, two caesareans normally means caesareans for all future babies.

Risks of caesareans

There is a slightly higher risk of maternal death and of infections after the operation. The mother needs time to recover from such a major operation, and this can be a problem with a new baby to look after, who may also be suffering from complications. It may be difficult to establish breastfeeding properly.

BREECH BABIES

Most babies have sorted out their final position by about thirty-four to thirty-six weeks. This is usually head first, the baby lying head down in the uterus. At forty weeks 3 per cent of babies are in the breech position. Your consultant will then want to discuss the various options with you. The baby can be born safely through the vagina bottom first as long as your pelvis is big enough. If there's any doubt, an X-ray of your pelvis may be arranged and a caesarean section done if it's too small or if the baby is lying in a particularly awkward position.

STILLBIRTH AND NEONATAL DEATH

Stillbirth – also called *intrauterine death* – occurs when the baby dies in the uterus and is born dead. A *neonatal death* occurs when the baby lives for less than a month. As many as 6000 babies are stillborn every year in this country and about the same number die after birth.

'Why me, why my baby?' are usually the first questions bereaved parents ask. A post mortem can help to find out why, and your consultant will want to speak to you after the post mortem to try to explain what happened.

You may feel angry with the hospital, that more could have been done; or you may feel guilty with yourself, perhaps for not coming to the hospital sooner. Your family doctor, midwife or health visitor are the best people to talk such things over with, giving you time to express yourself and helping with the reasons.

It's sometimes harder to get over having a stillborn baby than one that's lived for a while: the memories are mainly ones of looking forward to the baby's arrival, the planning and reorganisation of your lives. The grieving process and getting over it seem to be made easier by seeing and holding the baby after it's born. Some hospitals will also give you a photograph of your child, which can be a comfort later on. It can be hard when, in an effort to be kind and perhaps because they are feeling a bit uncomfortable as well, friends and relatives may not want to talk about it all – even though you do. Some suggest you should have another baby as soon as possible This is a decision for you and your partner to make; it's usually better to wait a while and mourn the baby and come to terms with the loss. Your doctor will be able to help you with this, advising you on any particular precautions to be taken.

Getting over the loss of a baby takes some time: the delivery date, your last period, when the baby died – these dates will continue to remind you as you start to live again. Tears and disappointment will be replaced in time with a feeling of sadness.

Stillbirth and Neonatal Death Society, 28 Portland Place, London W1N 4DE. Tel: 071–436 5881. They will provide further information and support.

INFERTILITY

Of normal healthy couples, 80 per cent will have conceived within a year of trying for a baby and 90 per cent within two years. This leaves one in ten couples with a problem. Most doctors are reluctant to do anything major in the way of investigations and treatment until at least one year has elapsed in case conception occurs naturally. For some people this waiting can be very frustrating and upsetting, especially when a woman has delayed having a baby because of a career or a second marriage. However, most doctors take a sympathetic view, and even more so when the women is in her thirties.

Seeking help with conception means you both have to face up to the problem. During the course of investigation and treatment you will be asked personal questions about your sex life, your partner will have to produce a semen specimen by masturbation, and you may be advised when and when not to have sex. You may have to travel distances to visit special clinics on a regular basis, and treatment can be a drain on your finances. It's a difficult journey to embark upon and can cause enough stress to threaten even the happiest and most secure of partnerships.

Before sending you to a gynaecologist, your family doctor may want to do some simple tests first. The following are some questions that need to be answered.

Are you both generally healthy?
Being either overweight or underweight will reduce your chances of conception, so will smoking.

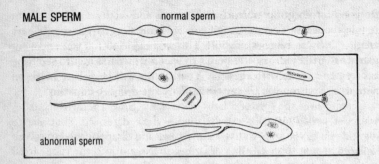

Thyroid disorders can have an effect on fertility, as can the more serious chronic illnesses, such as renal failure or auto-immune diseases. Viral infections such as flu can cause a drop in the sperm count. Certain drugs can do this too. Some men naturally have a low sperm count, and a third of infertility problems are due to this, so a semen test should be done early on. The semen is produced (usually at home by masturbation) and brought to the pathology laboratory for testing. The sperm will be counted, and their swimming potential assessed.

How often are you having sex?

Most doctors would expect you to be having intercourse somewhere in the region of two to three times a week to maximise the chance of conceiving. In an average menstrual cycle of twenty-eight days the egg is released on day fourteen and lives for about twenty-four hours. Sperms can live for several days, so sex around the middle of the month is likely to be the most successful. However, anxiety about when to have sex can be counter-productive – it's better to make love because you feel like it rather than because the calendar says so. Many doctors have abandoned the idea of getting women to take their temperature every day (body temperature goes up slightly at ovulation time) because of the anxiety created.

Some clinics offer a *post-coital test*, similar to taking a smear, where a sample of the cervical mucus is looked at under the microscope. This is done around the time of ovulation. You must have intercourse that day or the night before. A good result shows swimming sperms in the mucus, which indicates that the sperm are getting to the right place, and that the mucus is friendly and welcoming. If the mucus isn't right (wrong time of the month, or not ovulating regularly), then dead sperm or none at all will be seen.

Do you have regular periods?

Regular monthly periods usually mean normal egg production and release. This can be checked with a simple blood test. Drugs – often known as fertility drugs – are used to encourage ovulation if there is a problem and are quite successful. There is a small chance of twins or more, but most couples are very keen to try the drugs despite this.

Are your Fallopian tubes open?

The egg is fertilised in the tube by a sperm which has managed to travel from the vagina through the cervix and uterus up into the tube. It is essential, therefore, that this pathway is freely open for the sperm to reach the egg so that fertilisation can take place. The fertilised egg then needs to travel down to the uterus to embed and grow.

Problems with pelvic infections (chlamydia and gonorrhoea, pages 87 and 88) and inflammation (endometriosis, page 57) can cause scarring inside and outside the tubes and around the ovaries. There may be difficulty with egg release or with transport in the tube.

LAPAROSCOPY In such cases, a laparoscopy (page 47) is recommended. The ovaries, tubes and uterus are checked, and so are the supporting ligaments (a common site for endometriosis). It is possible to see the appearance of recent ovulation in the ovaries if this is the right time of the month. To check the tubes, dye is normally injected through the cervix. If the tubes are open, the dye can be seen through the laparoscope spilling out of the frond-like ends of the tubes (fimbriae). The dye is passed from the vagina afterwards.

HYSTEROSALPINGOGRAM (HSG) Some doctors prefer to check if the tubes are open with an X-ray (a *hysterosalpingogram*, or HSG). You are usually awake for this. First you are examined as for a smear test with a speculum (page 30), then the dye is injected through the cervix. Some women find this uncomfortable (ask your doctor about pain relief beforehand), but it's over fairly rapidly.

What treatments are available?

Endometriosis is quite a common finding in women with infertility. Treatment is lengthy (six months to a year) and stops ovulation and menstruation. Drugs used are danazol (Danol tablets) and buserilin (Suprefact, a nasal spray), which prevent the monthly stimulation of the uterus lining. Success rates following treatment are very variable.

INFERTILITY DRUGS Clomiphene citrate, taken as tablets, is commonly used. It may over-stimulate the ovaries. This is sometimes combined with the hormone human chorionic gonadotrophin (HCG), which helps the egg to release. You can experience tiredness, headaches and mood changes.

Human menopausal gonadotrophin (HMG) is a powerful hormone (Pergonal), and is usually only used when all else has failed. This contains FSH and LH hormones, which induce ovulation. Again, care must be taken that the ovaries are not over-stimulated.

Hypothalamic releasing factors involve pumping the hormone LHRH (the hormone that enables LH to be released) in small, short bursts (an easy portable pump is worn for this). This mimics the natural release of the hormone in the body. Ultrasound scanning of the ovaries is frequently done with these treatments to check the development of the eggs. Trans-vaginal scanning, where a small probe is inserted into the vagina, is a new technique which shows the ovaries very clearly.

ARTIFICIAL INSEMINATION This is considered when either the husband is fertile but impotent, or the man is infertile and donor semen available. Donated sperm is transferred into the vagina using a syringe, usually for the three or four days around ovulation. It is not widely available on the NHS, and private clinics can be expensive, in which case the charity BPAS may be your best bet. The donor must be properly screened, and complete anonymity assured. You should think carefully before going ahead with AI, and counselling may help – what will you tell family and friends, what will you tell the child?

SURGERY If the tubes are blocked, or there are other structural problems of the uterus, then surgery is usually the first treatment. However, even using the most careful microscopic technique, the success rate in terms of getting pregnant and having a healthy baby is no more than 50 per cent. As laser surgery becomes more common, there may be a higher success rate.

IN-VITRO FERTILISATION (IVF) If your tubes are damaged, assisted conception (in-vitro fertilisation, IVF) may be necessary. Only a few centres around the country offer this within the NHS, but there are many private clinics available. If you're considering going to a private clinic make sure it's one your consultant recommends. She will need to write to them with your details to save repeating all the tests.

IVF is primarily suitable for women with damaged or absent Fallopian tubes (perhaps due to ectopic pregnancies in the past). Couples with other sorts of infertility may also be suitable (low sperm count, endometriosis), as will couples with no apparent causes for infertility. After thorough checking of your details and investigations you will both be counselled about the procedure, its success rate – about 25 per cent – and the risks of multiple pregnancy.

The ovaries are stimulated with hormones (Pergonal, Humegon) so that more than one egg develops. Just before ovulation the eggs are 'harvested': retrieved either through a laparoscope (you have to be asleep) or by a needle in the vagina guided by an ultrasound scan (you're awake but sedated). The eggs are checked for quality, mixed with your partner's specially prepared sperm, and then placed in an incubator where they start to grow. The fertilised eggs (no more than three normally) are put into the uterus through a fine tube about three or four days later. This is a quick, painless procedure.

Another method is *gamete* (meaning the sperm or egg) *intra fallopian transfer* (GIFT). The eggs are again produced using hormones, then mixed with the sperm and placed back in the Fallopian tube through a laparoscope (page 47). Fertilisation takes place naturally. The success rate for this is higher – about 30 per cent – but it is not suitable if your tubes are blocked or scarred, or if you have already had an ectopic pregnancy.

The tests show nothing wrong – what now?
Sadly, a large proportion of infertile couples have nothing physically wrong with them. Sometimes, in such cases, the problem may be psychological. Has either of you been suffering from stress, or depresssion or anxiety? Have you suffered a long-term trauma? The whole process of trying for a baby – the tests, unspontaneous sex, failure – can also cause mental tensions. Psychotherapy or counselling may help in such instances. For others, it may be easier to come to terms with the fact that they will never get pregnant rather than dealing with the constant anxiety and pressure of trying. Some couples have found that once they 'let go', everything has sorted itself out on its own. Often this happens on holiday, or at the start of a new job, just those times when you have other things on your mind.

> *We tried for a child for five years. We didn't worry about it, and my husband and I didn't really talk about it because we were afraid, I suppose, that one of us might have a problem.*
>
> *Then we decided to go and see a doctor together – he sent us to the infertility unit in Bristol – they talked to us – asked us both about our life history, about our families, and whether or not there had been any cases of infertility in either of our families. They gave us*

both a test. In those days they didn't have as much knowledge as they do now, and I think they did a lot more tests than they needed to. I spent four years going back and forward from the unit, having tests. I got very tired, sometimes I would have to go once a week. It got difficult at work because I couldn't tell my boss where I was going. It was stressful.

They didn't find anything. They gave me various tablets including fertility tablets for about a year. I had a gland at the back of my neck which they tested thinking maybe it was stress related. They did tests on my husband's sperm and my eggs. They put the sperm and eggs with others, but concluded that if anything our eggs and sperm were more compatible together, the best combination.

I got to know a female doctor very well who I felt comfortable with – she encouraged us but didn't pressurise us. She actually lead us to give up smoking which was a good thing – sometimes smoking can hinder fertility.

I was given the chance to have IVF on the NHS which I took. It's where they recover any eggs and mix them with my husband's sperm. It didn't work the first time, they found I had traces of endometriosis. I was put on Danol tablets for 4–5 months. Because of that problem I was entitled to go through IVF again. I went through it again, with no luck.

I had no more chances with the NHS. I went private this year; because I was made redundant, I decided to use my redundancy money on GIFT (test tube baby).

GIFT is like IVF, but more natural, it's the same process but they mix the egg with the sperm straight away, and put three eggs back in through the Fallopian tubes. This didn't work. I still have 4 eggs frozen at the clinic, but if I wanted to try again it would cost hundreds of pounds just to get the eggs de-frosted.

Now at thirty-eight, I've decided to try naturally over the next two years. I've bought an ovulation kit from the NHS, which tells you when is the best time. I go to a herbalist regularly. I've decided to get my body healthy.

Women's Health, 52 Featherstone Street, London EC1Y 8RT. Tel: 071–251 6580.

—5—
AFTER THE BIRTH

Getting back to normal after having a baby is a little like recovering from an operation, except that you have a small demanding bundle who doesn't know the difference between day and night and is always hungry and it's yours. It's very easy to focus on the baby and forget to look after yourself. However difficult the first few months are, remember to leave some time for yourself and you and your partner.

EARLY DAYS

Most women stay in hospital for between two and five days to get some rest, especially if they have young families at home. This also gives breastfeeding mothers a chance to get the feeding sorted out before going home. Once at home, your local midwife will visit you for at least ten days, followed by the health visitor. This means there's lots of help and support available in the early days.

YOUR EMOTIONS Most women feel in a complete turmoil the first few days: cloud nine one minute, the depths of despair the next – this is due to the hormones plummeting back to normal. The majority of women recognise the third day blues (although it's more likely to be the fourth or fifth) where everything is just too much, there are tears at the slightest upset, and you wonder how on earth you will ever manage. It's hard enough to cope with this new responsibility when you're 100 per cent fit; it can be overwhelming when you are feeling tired and sore, perhaps struggling to breastfeed, in a relatively strange environment.

Most women find themselves on a more even keel after they have been back home for a week or so.

YOUR BODY Unfortunately, your abdomen doesn't shrink back to its normal size straight away, so you'll still look pregnant. Over the next fourteen days it will improve until your midwife won't be able to feel the uterus through your abdomen. The rest is up to you and exercise.

VAGINAL BLEEDING AND PERIODS After the baby is born, you will experience quite a heavy blood loss (lochia) over the first few days (you'll need good size sanitary pads) which gradually settles down to a lighter brownish loss. It may increase as you get more mobile, but should in general be lessening as the days go by. Most women stop bleeding soon after two weeks, some continue for a month (particularly those who have had babies already), and then it merges with a normal period. Use sanitary pads until the first period. Bleeding carrying on after this or if the loss gets heavy with clots must be reported to your midwife, as should any low abdominal pain or unpleasant odour from the loss. Any of these symptoms may mean a small piece of placenta has remained in the uterus and become infected. You may need antibiotics and a D & C type operation (evacuation of the uterus, page 50) to make sure the uterus is empty.

Some women have a period as soon as four weeks after the birth. Other mothers, usually the ones who are breastfeeding, may not see a period for as long as six months (but don't forget that you can get pregnant before you have a period). After the first baby your uterus will be slightly larger, and you may find your periods are a little heavier. Tampons may not fit as well if you've had an episiotomy or a tear; by four to six weeks it's okay to use them, but you may need sanitary pads as well for the heavy days.

YOUR BLADDER It may be quite difficult to pass urine in the first few hours after the baby is born, especially if you've had an epidural or an episiotomy. If you can't pass urine, your midwife will drain the bladder for you with a catheter tube. This procedure doesn't hurt and the relief is enormous.

The bladder soon comes back to normal, but you may find you have little control at first. Coughing and laughing may make you leak. Tell the midwife; sometimes this can mean that the urine is infected. It is a reminder to keep doing your pelvic floor exercises – practise stopping and starting in the middle of your flow of urine (page 150). It may seem impossible at first, but the pelvic power soon comes back.

YOUR BOWELS If you've had an episiotomy the stitches are very close to your bottom. Passing a motion for the first time can be a little sore, but don't worry about the stitches, they won't come out; holding a sanitary pad against the stitches makes it more comfortable. Avoid straining if you can. Keep constipation at bay by eating a high roughage diet (not always available in hospital) and get your partner to bring in high fibre foods that work for you. It may be more difficult to keep your bottom clean, especially if you've got a problem with piles. Use moistened tissues (baby wipes) as well as toilet paper.

YOUR BREASTS They will feel heavier and tingly on the second day as the milk prepares to flow. You will probably be more comfortable wearing a bra all the time, even in bed. Make sure it's a good supporting bra for nursing purposes.

If you're not planning to breastfeed the milk will dry up on its own. If there's no one suckling the message will get through that the milk is not required and the production will stop. The breasts may be uncomfortable while this is happening – firm bra support and analgesics (paracetamol) are helpful.

GETTING COMFORTABLE After my first baby I remember feeling I had pads everywhere – nipples, breasts, sanitary towels. Walking was difficult – I felt as though a horse had kicked my bottom and my back ached from the epidural. Lying in the bath with milk dripping from my breasts, I craved to be normal again.

It may be difficult to walk upright and sit straight after an episiotomy or a caesarean section. Make an effort to avoid tensing your muscles as much as possible, in particular the shoulders. When you're sitting to feed the baby, make sure you're comfortable first. Sit on a ring (a rubber inflatable one) or cushion, with your arms well supported, and in such a way that you are able to rest your head back. Don't rush, settle yourself down even if the baby's crying; feeding will be much more enjoyable for you both if you're comfortable.

ESSENTIAL EXERCISE

As the uterus shrinks back to its normal shape and you start moving around, the muscles in the pelvis and abdomen will regain their tone. To help this along start off actively exercising in hospital.

UTERUS AFTER BIRTH

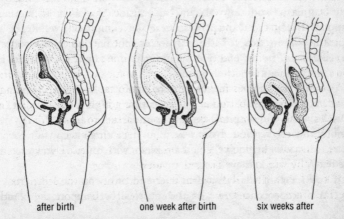

after birth   one week after birth   six weeks after

149

Abdominal muscle exercises Before you take on anything more vigorous, try lying on your back with your knees bent up and breathe deeply. As you breathe in let your abdomen rise, then breathe out, firmly pulling in your tummy muscles. Repeat this six times.

Still in the same position, place your hands on the front of your thighs. Lift up your head and neck and reach your hands down towards your knees. Count to three and relax. You should feel your muscles pulling. Repeat this exercise six times. Try and do both of these exercises every hour.

You may be given further instructions on abdominal exercises in hospital, but don't be too enthusiastic and do too much too quickly. The ligaments supporting your pelvis and back are still soft and vulnerable from your increased hormone levels. They are much easier to damage in the early days.

Pelvic Floor Muscles All exercise indirectly strengthens the pelvic floor; but it is essential to do specific pelvic exercises. The vagina and supporting ligaments of the uterus are greatly stretched by pregnancy and childbirth. These same ligaments also support the bladder and rectum; if they're weak, there's the danger you could wet yourself when you cough or sneeze. Prolapse of the uterus occurs when the supporting ligaments are so weakened that the cervix and uterus come down the vagina (you may feel a lump, you may just get a dragging feeling).

Getting the vagina back to normal is also important for enjoying sex again for you and your partner.

You can do pelvic floor exercises sitting, lying or standing up – no one knows you're doing them. Concentrate on closing your anus as though you were trying to stop passing wind. At the same time draw your vagina in and upwards and squeeze, as if closing in around a tampon. If you can, hold this squeeze for a count of five. Relax and repeat four more times. Then start again, but now hold for a count of one each time. By the end, you should have done five long squeezes and five short squeezes.

You may feel at first after having the baby that nothing is happening at all. Keep exercising and as the days pass you will begin to feel the muscles move and you may be able to squeeze for longer. Ideally, you should aim to do these every hour, but four times a day is probably more realistic to begin with, perhaps when you're sitting down feeding the baby. Try to do them as often as you remember.

If you are particularly worried about incontinence of urine, make a special effort to concentrate on the muscles that support the bladder.

When you are passing urine practise stopping and starting before you've actually finished; interrupting the flow in this way is an excellent way of exercising these muscles.

These exercises are for life. Ideally, we should teach our daughters to do them from childhood to ensure they don't suffer from these particular problems later on.

BONDING – IS IT A MYTH?

What if you don't actually love your baby? Some mothers fall in love with their babies straight away; others find it takes time to get to know the baby and develop a protective maternal instinct.

The bonding theory was first proposed in the early 1970s when research stressed the importance of establishing a good mother–baby relationship. This has left some women feeling confused and guilty, because they didn't experience intense love for their babies right from the beginning. Recent research has shown, however, that as many as 40 per cent of mothers don't feel this initial wave of love. Many didn't feel particularly strongly about the baby until the fourth or fifth day. Bonding is an ongoing process, so don't feel guilty if you take longer to settle down with your baby.

There's no magic about bonding; mothers who are separated from their babies in Special Care, for example, have to adjust to the situation and usually make up for lost time when the baby comes home. Couples who adopt babies or toddlers rarely find difficulty in loving their children, despite missing out on the first weeks or months of life.

Learning to love your baby is like developing any new relationship. You'll soon work out what your baby likes and doesn't like, and the baby soon realises you're her main source of nourishment, comfort and affection.

Part of the problem may be that most couples feel inhibited within the hospital setting. If the midwife leaves you and your partner and the baby alone for a while soon after the birth, take the opportunity to enjoy contact with the baby – kissing and cuddling and exploring her body. This is as important for your partner as it is for you.

FEEDING THE BABY

Breastfeeding is best for the baby and you, but at the moment probably only one in four babies are receiving their mother's milk: full of goodness, absolutely fresh, additive free, ridiculously cheap and extremely convenient.

What's so special about breast milk?

Unlike cow's milk, which is designed for calves, breast milk contains all the right ingredients to feed and nourish your baby for at least six months. It gives your baby antibodies in the precious early weeks before the baby can make her own. This protects against coughs and colds and stomach troubles. Breast milk may also help prevent or delay the development of allergy problems, such as asthma and eczema. Breastfed babies usually put on just the right amount of weight, too, but don't worry if the baby seems overweight: the baby will lose this as soon as crawling starts. It comes out at the right temperature, on demand, and germ free. And if the baby needs more, more will be produced.

Breastfeeding is enjoyable for you and the baby. It gives you a wonderful feeling of closeness, helps bonding, and there is also the satisfaction and pleasure in providing food so naturally for the baby. It is also supposed to help the mother regain her pre-pregnant shape more easily, but I'm afraid I don't believe it. I didn't find this to be the case, and research has shown that our metabolic rate slows down when we are breastfeeding and we conserve our fat stores for the baby.

What's so wrong with bottle feeding?

With all these very good reasons for breastfeeding, mothers who can't manage it may feel incredibly guilty. Midwives are taught to encourage and support women with breastfeeding, so if things aren't going well they may react negatively to a move to the bottle. You may end up feeling confused and a failure.

Formula milks are modified cow's milk, altered to mimic breast milk ingredients (this means reducing the amount of protein and salt found in cow's milk). There are two main hazards with bottle feeding. The first is the greater risk of infection of the stomach and bowel (gastro-enteritis). Great care is needed with sterilising bottles and teats for this reason. The second is that if the feeds are not carefully made up, there is a danger that the baby may have either a too concentrated or too diluted feed. The result may look like a digestive upset, but can go on to be quite dangerous for the baby.

Is there anything good about bottle feeding? Yes: you can share it with your partner; you can have a night's sleep if he's prepared to do the occasional night for you; and you can go out together if you have a reliable babysitter. (You can, of course, express your milk too.) Some mothers feel it's helpful to know how much milk the baby's getting. They can work out the baby's intake from day to day.

How to breastfeed

The vast majority of women (97 per cent) are physically capable of breastfeeding their babies successfully. The size and shape of your breasts and nipples have nothing to do with being good at breastfeeding. Your chances of success are much more dependent on the baby being correctly positioned on the breast.

Research has shown that babies fed within the first thirty minutes of birth are more likely to be breastfed for longer. Early physical contact with the baby seems to help, too.

Being successful with the first feed starts things off on a very good footing. But you must remember that breastfeeding is a skill to be learned and practised; it's not instinctive. Even second- or third-time mothers often need help in getting started, especially if there have been problems before.

Don't restrict feeds, the baby alone knows when she's had enough. Babies who are fed when they want gain weight quicker and are usually breastfed for longer.

Night feeds, although a shock to the system, form a large part of the baby's calorie intake. Giving the baby a bottle of milk at night will reduce your milk supply. In fact, breastfeeding at night gives milk production an extra boost.

National Childbirth Trust, Breastfeeding Promotion Group, Alexandra House, Oldham Terrace, London W3 6NH. Tel: 081–992 8637 for further information.

La Leche League, Breastfeeding Help and Information, BM3424, London WC1N 3XX. Tel: 071–242 1278.

Association of Breast Feeding Mothers, 10 Herschell Road, London SE23. Tel: 081–778 4769.

THE EARLY WEEKS

Life was so easy before, now you have to do everything you did before *and* look after an unpredictable baby. Enjoying a quiet cup of coffee may seem like a dream in the early days. It's important to get your priorities right at this stage. Let the housework slide – friends are coming to see you and the new baby, not admire the dusting. Try to arrange for some extra help in the house for the first few weeks; you may be entitled to a home help for a short period (ask the local Social Services department). If you have a partner and he is entitled to take paternity leave, great; if not, he will probably want to take ordinary holiday to help you get sorted out at the beginning. Remember, motherhood is not an instinct that suddenly appears when the baby is born: it has to be learnt like any other skill.

If you're finding it really difficult to cope, ask a friend to whip round and tidy up while you make the coffee. It'll make you feel better. Most important is to have someone to listen to you and to get a bit of sympathy. If you are stuck without any family nearby or close friends, your midwife, who will be visiting you at home, may be able to help. The local NCT group can also be very useful; they should be able to put you in touch with other mothers.

SLEEPING Be ruthless about getting some sleep. This may not be easy if you're breastfeeding, but some mothers express milk in advance so that their partners can feed the baby once in a while. If you're bottle feeding, don't hesitate to share the feeding when your partner is around and available.

You will soon find your baby has some kind of routine after the first week; there will be times of quite prolonged sleep (often in the morning), which is the best time for you to have a nap as well. Warn your midwife and friends, and take the phone off the hook if you like.

During the night it's not always necessary for you to change the baby's nappy if it's not dirty – this saves needlessly disrupting you or the baby. It's thought that breastfeeding actually makes a woman feel sleepy by producing the brain chemical *dopamine* together with the breastfeeding hormone *oxytocin*. This enables you to get back to sleep quickly at night.

If the baby's cot is right next to you, the easiest way to feed the baby is in bed with you. If this disturbs your partner, sleep in separate beds until the baby is more settled. There seems to be no evidence that having the baby sleeping in bed with you is either harmful or dangerous and it may be the only solution to settling a disturbed baby. To do this safely both parents and baby must be healthy: it can be dangerous if either parent is ill, sedated, drunk or very overweight. It's best to make sure there is some barrier at the edge of the bed to prevent the baby accidentally rolling out.

EATING AND LOSING WEIGHT It's probably best to forget the weight and the waist in the early days. There's so much going on that you'll be lucky to get a decent meal yourself. Try to avoid high calorie snacks which seem so tempting when you're tired; limit yourself to perhaps one packet of crisps, or a small chocolate bar a day to keep your spirits up. A sandwich is just as good as a cooked meal.

Serious slimming should wait until the baby is three months old, has settled into a routine and is giving you a reasonably good night's sleep. Although much is made of breastfeeding assisting weight loss, it actually slows down the metabolic rate to ensure reserves are kept for the baby. Some women find the weight impossible to lose until they stop breastfeeding.

SEX – WHEN? Most women start to have sex again when the vaginal loss settles (page 147). If you've had an episiotomy, it's best to wait for three to four weeks for it to heal. If you're in any doubt, wait until your six-week postnatal visit.

The first time you make love after the baby is born will be a little sore, so take it slowly and use a lubricating jelly (KY) if it helps.

CONTRACEPTION

It's a good idea to have thought about contraception and discussed it with the hospital staff before you go home, feel you have the weight of the world on your shoulders and an accident happens.

ORAL CONTRACEPTION If you're bottle feeding, you may well ovulate again within a few weeks (usually two weeks before your period starts). If you were taking the combined oral contraceptive Pill you can go back on this. Most doctors advise you start the Pill on the first day of your first period to avoid taking extra oestrogens while your own body levels are still on the high side (danger of thrombosis). If you have intercourse before this use a condom.

If you're breastfeeding, high levels of the pituitary hormone *prolactin* will switch your ovaries off. This is not entirely reliable and becomes less so if the feeds are supplemented with cow's milk or the baby is being weaned. The progestogen-only Pill (Mini-pill) is recommended if you want oral contraception and plan to breastfeed. The combined Pill is an unnecessarily strong contraceptive when lactation is doing most of its work. The combined Pill also reduces the volume and quality of the milk. You can start the progestogen-only Pill straight away (although some doctors advise a wait of seven days). Minute quantities of the hormone do get into the breast milk, but blood tests on the babies have failed to show any hormone at all in their circulation. This Pill has no effect on the quality of the breast milk.

IUD This can be fitted at your postnatal visit; use a condom if you have sex before this.

DIAPHRAGM If you used a diaphragm before your pregnancy it must be checked afterwards. Your internal and external dimensions may well have changed, and you could be more than 3 kg/7 lb heavier than pre-pregnancy. You will then need a new diaphragm fitted.

THE POSTNATAL VISIT
The postnatal visit normally takes place when the baby is six weeks old. It may be combined with a check on the baby at the same time.

Write down in advance anything that's worrying you – when you get there and the baby decides she needs a feed or makes a large mess on the bed, you may completely forget what you wanted to say.

The doctor will ask you details about your lochia (vaginal loss) and whether you've had a period yet. Contraception will be discussed if you've not sorted it out already. Your doctor will also want to know if you're having sex and, if so, whether there are any problems.

A blood pressure and urine check are done. Your abdomen is examined – the doctor shouldn't be able to feel the uterus at this stage. A pelvic examination of the uterus will be done to make sure it's back to the right size, and any episiotomy or tear scar looked at; say if you're finding it uncomfortable. A cervical smear can be taken now if it's due.

If you're having problems with leaking urine or a dragging feeling in the vagina after standing, your doctor will emphasise the importance of doing your pelvic floor exercises again and again (page 150). Keep working on them, they really will make a difference.

If you've had a difficult delivery – a caesarean section or a forceps delivery – discuss the reasons with your doctor. This may well not happen next time but sometimes a repeat caesarean section is advised. Most decisions like these, however, are usually made in the next pregnancy by your consultant obstetrician.

REGISTRATION AND BENEFITS
You have six weeks after the delivery within which to register the baby and get a birth certificate. (This can be extended in exceptional circumstances.) Some units arrange for the Registrar to come to the hospital which can be quite convenient if you've decided on the baby's name. Once the baby is registered, you can claim child benefit (a form will be given to you to fill in and send off). You can choose how you want the benefit to be paid: weekly, monthly or paid into a separate account. You may also be eligible for family credit if your partner earns less than a certain amount.

Prescriptions and dental treatment remain free for you for the first year of the baby's life.

THE FUTURE

FEELINGS AND RELATIONSHIPS

Changing from being just the two of you to a new life revolving around a baby needs a lot of readjustment for you both.

Many new mothers feel depressed and unable to cope in the first few months. They can feel inadequate and a failure, particularly if breastfeeding isn't going well. It's normal to feel a need to be mothered yourself, too. Women who have held down demanding jobs before the birth, and coped wonderfully with working and the pregnancy, may come down to earth with a bump when they feel they can't even manage looking after a baby. A mother can also easily feel neglected and think that no one is interested in her problems when midwives and health visitors, friends and relations are all focused on the baby. In a recent study with depressed mothers, health visitors were asked to include half-an-hour's counselling for the mother with each visit. These mothers reported the visits much more helpful and supportive. More and more health workers are realising that in these days when your mother doesn't live round the corner and you may not even know your neighbours, the framework of reassuring support isn't always there, and they are doing their best to help mothers at one of the most stressful times in their lives.

Keep in touch with the mothers at your parentcraft class or find out about your local NCT group for moral support and sympathy. Babies are also welcome at mother and toddler groups, and these are a good way to meet other mothers in the area. If you feel nervous about going or need help with the baby, get a friend to come with you the first time.

Some women find themselves missing being pregnant. Pregnancy for some acts as an escape from the harsh realities of the world: jobs they don't really like, unemployment, fending for themselves. When the baby arrives it's back to the real world. Some women find themselves thinking nostalgically of those pregnant days, when they were made to feel special. They lose the exclusively close relationship with the baby inside – some women still imagine they feel the baby kicking for a while, some long for those quiet serene days of pregnancy.

Your partner Although it's expected these days for your partner to be with you in labour, being the 'new man', perhaps half of them feel out of place. Going to parentcraft classes with you and learning how to support and care for you in labour will give him the confidence to be there right from the beginning.

Men in our society aren't particularly encouraged to do the nurturing and enjoy spending time with the baby. Their role is to do the jobs; they're back to work, or helping in the house and doing the shopping. Because of this it can take longer for a man to form a strong relationship with the baby, and he may feel nervous if left in charge. However, he does need to be given time and space to be responsible for the baby sometimes, without you or others interfering. He has to work out the baby's personality for himself and start to interact and love her. Your partner, too, may be feeling jealous of the baby for taking your attention away from him. As the pregnancy has progressed you will both have subtly altered your lifestyles in preparation for the new baby. There'll have been less socialising, less alcohol, and more of the nesting, such as decorating and helping with the domestic chores. Once the baby has arrived, your partner will have to be prepared to lend a hand, make do with simple meals or cook them himself, and generally be aware of what you're up against. At the same time, try not to forget his needs: the disturbed nights will make him tired, too; he will want to relax when he comes home from work as usual, even if you're desperate to park the baby with him. He may have missed out on the sexual side of your relationship for quite a while; remember to be affectionate and loving even if you're too tired to respond physically.

Can having a baby ruin your sex life?

Most couples find it difficult re-establishing a sex life after the birth of a baby. For some, this can take up to two or three years. Having a baby takes a period of adjustment for both parents; sometimes this appears as a loss of interest in sex by the woman.

Most people don't openly talk in depth about their sexual diffi-culties, so it's hard to know if what we are feeling is normal and to be expected, or if something's wrong.

THE VAGINA Poorly repaired episiotomies and tears are responsible for making intercourse sore and uncomfortable. Stitches should be dis-solved and the wound healed by the time the baby is four weeks old. Many women wait until their six-week check before giving intercourse a try. Take things slowly at first – the area just at the entrance many still be tender – and use a lubricating jelly (KY). Persistence with intercourse will help to stretch the vaginal tissues, so it should get easier and easier. If it doesn't, tell your doctor; there may be one spot of raw tissue that's not healed. Your doctor can cauterise this by applying a tiny bit of silver nitrate. If the repair has healed poorly in general it may be as well to have this redone in hospital (usually an overnight stay, done under general anaesthetic). If you can't face intercourse because of the pain you're better off seeking help.

Once the perineum has been stretched the vagina isn't so effective as a container. You may find semen leaks out after intercourse uncontrollably, as does the start of a period. Also, as the seal isn't so effective, its easier for air to enter the vagina during intercourse, which can mean passing wind at the height of passion. This can result in deep embarrassment or a fit of the giggles. Change your intercourse position if this is a problem. Pelvic floor exercises may improve it (page 150).

EXHAUSTION In the first few weeks, when it's normal to feel exceptionally tired, it's hardly surprising that sex takes a back seat. Try going to bed early, as soon as the baby has been fed, and take your partner with you. Just lying together – holding each other and chatting over what's happened during the day – may relax you both and get you in the mood. If it doesn't just enjoy the break and being together.

YOUR HORMONES Breastfeeding switches your ovaries off, so the amount of oestrogen in your body drops, sometimes to the levels reached in the menopause. This can make your vagina dry and poorly lubricated during sex, causing discomfort. A lubricating jelly (KY) will help, or an oestrogen cream from your doctor if it doesn't. Because your hormones are low, there aren't the monthly surges which make some women very interested in sex.

BODY SHAPE New mothers are very vulnerable to anything that can shatter their confidence. They're worried about coping with the baby: are they doing right with feeding, clothing, caring? A woman may look at herself and think: what on earth do I look like? If she always made an effort to look good and dress well, she may be quite depressed with her new image. Still in maternity or baggy clothes, no figure to speak of, too tired to apply make-up, her image of herself as a confident sexually attractive woman goes out of the window.

It's important not to worry; your figure will work itself out with a sensible diet and regular exercise, and as you settle down to a routine with the baby you must start to find more time for yourself.

TOO MUCH LOVE? There is a danger that the new relationship a mother has with her baby ends up excluding her partner. She may well replace sex with the physical expression of love for the baby and any other children. It may not always be apparent to you that this is going on, but it's worth thinking about. Let your partner hold and play with the baby in the evenings, even if it's the best time of the day as far as the baby's mood goes. Get a baby sitter occasionally and go out as a couple again; it can do you both the world of good and may make you feel more relaxed.

WORRY ABOUT THE BABY If the baby is born prematurely or if there's a problem at birth, your first few weeks, and maybe months, may be spent in a relentless state of stress and worry. Sex can be ignored; you may feel you're not allowed to enjoy yourself when the baby is unwell. Talk together, tell each other what your problems and worries are. Keep communicating during the difficult time; sex may even be a help in relieving the tension.

The best relationships are put under enormous strain when a baby arrives. Keeping the lines of communication open is the most important thing of all. Tell each other how you feel, and work out a survival plan in the knowledge that things do get better.

If you have a problem your family doctor can refer you to a psychosexual clinic – most cities have a service. Your local Relate (Marriage Guidance) group may offer help (look them up in your local phone directory).

British Association of Sexual and Marital Therapists, PO Box 62, Sheffield, S10 3TS. Send s.a.e. for further information.

POSTNATAL DEPRESSION AND ILLNESS
The emotional upset that hits most women in the first week of the baby's life passes quickly and life settles down. But for one in ten women the readjustment to a different life with the strain of a new baby, perhaps with little outside help, an untidy house, a confused or distant partner, can be very difficult and she becomes depressed. Half of these women will need medical help to get over this depression.

The symptoms are mood changes, frequently feeling tearful, feelings of inadequacy and not being able to cope. You may be off your food, off sex, and even when you get the chance find difficulty in sleeping.

Who gets depressed?
I'm sure all new mothers get depressed to some extent, but true postnatal depression is more common in certain types of women: those who were particularly anxious or depressed in pregnancy; mothers who have a difficult labour and delivery; single mothers; and those going through other family trauma like bereavement at the time of the birth.

Does it affect the baby?

Babies are highly sensitive to the quality of care they receive. When they're two weeks old they actually know and prefer their caretaker's voice and smell. A depressed mother doesn't respond to her baby anywhere near as much as a happy one, the relationship is affected and the baby becomes discontented in general. This may then affect the interaction between mother and baby for months to come.

Health care workers are trying to improve ways of picking up the problem before it does start to affect the whole family. In some areas a questionnaire has been developed giving the mother space to express her feelings.

Your doctor will want to know that simple measures like counselling, going to a support group, arranging extra help in the house, have all been tried before resorting to antidepressant drugs or referral to a psychiatrist.

PUERPERAL PSYCHOSIS

This is the name given to the much rarer, serious mental illness that affects between one in 500 and one in 1000 women each year. It happens more often to first-time mothers. Bizarre manic behaviour is noticed within a fornight of the baby's birth – it's thought to be due to the rapid drop in the hormone oestrogen level soon after the birth. This drop makes the dopamine system in the brain overactive, which triggers the symptoms of psychosis: euphoria, severe depression, hearing voices, feeling persecuted, and even wanting to harm the baby.

For safety's sake the mother has to be in hospital (the baby can usually come too) and drug treatment (tranquillisers like Largactil) and ECT (*electro convulsive therapy*) may be necessary. Some women respond quickly, others don't feel right for maybe a year.

Having had this frightening experience once, is it going to happen again? The risk is much greater than for the general population, but the chances seemed to be reduced if your partner is a good communicator, allowing time for discussion and talking over any worries, during the next pregnancy.

> *It began with anxiety. I went to the shops to get vegetables, and suddenly I couldn't stand it there any longer; a panic attack. I rushed out of the shop, heart pounding, I felt 'I can't cope'. That night I went to the doctor, a sympathetic friend had to accompany*

me, which is totally out of character for me. The doctor prescribed mild tranquillisers, which was fair enough but only for two weeks. They had no effect, and I began to have more and more panic attacks; I would wake up at 4.00 in the morning, just lie there worrying, heart thumping. You believe you might die. It was like being in a dentist's waiting room, waiting for major treatment but never getting treatment.

My husband was very sympathetic, and mother helped, too, but in a whole year nobody ever said I might be suffering from post-natal depression. One morning my husband had to come home from work, the doctor was called out and he gave me a course of anti-depressants. I went to bed for a week, but it took two weeks for the pills to work. I couldn't bear to see the children for more than five or ten minutes.

I limped along feeling up and down, but more down than up, for another four months and then I had another collapse like at the beginning. I went to see a psychiatrist, who took my whole case history. He immediately quadrupled the tablets and told me I'd be feeling better in three weeks. I didn't believe him at the time, but he was right. Three weeks later I woke up one morning and I knew instantly that I was OK again.

I had to stay on the drugs for a few more months but since then I really am back to my old self. None of it makes sense, I wanted the baby, in fact he was planned, there's no family history of depression, and I've had crises before but never reacted like this.

Looking back on the whole thing I feel a sense of loss, a loss of me and my skills. I distinctly remember I couldn't even decide to cut up some carrots I'd just peeled and stood crying in the kitchen.

Association for Post-Natal Illness, 25 Jerdan Place, Fulham, London SW6. Tel: 071–386 0868.

—6—

CHANGE FOR THE
BETTER

The physical changes of the menopause happen at a challenging time in a woman's life. Menopause means the end of menstruation. All that happens around this time is called the change of life (*climacteric*). She may have spent the last twenty years looking after the family, or developing a career or both, with not a minute to spare. Now, if there are children, they will probably have grown up and be in the process of leaving home, maybe with grandchildren in the offing. Elderly parents may add an extra strain. Her partner may be coming to terms with the reality of his career with its limitations, perhaps even redundancy.

This is quite enough stress without the odd hot flush and broken night. If you need help at this time consider talking to your family doctor. Menopause clinics are starting up in various parts of the country with specially trained staff to deal with menopause problems.

Try to keep occupied, take up new interests and meet new friends. Make the effort to get yourself out. Taking regular exercise is an excellent reason to join a keep fit class or swimming club.

What's happening inside?
The ovaries, after years of producing eggs, start to resist the effects of the pituitary hormones (*gonadotrophins*). They simply start to give up — sometimes producing an egg, sometimes not — and in the long run reducing the amounts of sex hormones released. The levels of oestrogen go down and the pituitary hormones increase in an effort to make the ovary work. A blood test measuring your gonadotrophin level can tell whether the menopause has arrived or is imminent.

When will the menopause start?
Most women stop their periods somewhere between the ages of forty-five and fifty-five, usually as a gradual process. The average age is fifty-one. Smokers stop their periods earlier, as do left-handed women.

There's no evidence to back up the well-known belief that the earlier your periods start the later they'll finish (or vice versa). It is true that women who've never been pregnant generally start the menopause earlier than those who've had children.

Will I survive?

Of course! Understanding what's going on is half the battle; knowing there's help if you need it is the rest.

Four out of five women get some symptoms due to low oestrogen levels, half of these suffer severely.

Certain changes, like hot flushes and sleep problems (see below), seem to be related to the sudden fall in hormones. Others, like vaginal dryness (page 165) and thinning bones, happen slowly as the body misses oestrogen (page 166). In the run up to the menopause the changing hormones may upset your period pattern: they may be lighter, they could well be very heavy.

Your mother's change may be a guide as to how you'll be, but don't forget treatment has greatly improved since then.

If you're fit and keep yourself occupied and interested, the menopause will not seem anywhere near so important, and remember you can do a lot to help yourself.

As your oestrogen levels go down so does the collagen in your skin. This can mean dry, flaky skin, dry hair, hair loss and brittle nails. Nobody has proved that losing your oestrogen supply prematurely gives you early wrinkles.

Some women have trouble with their gums and teeth; gingivitis is more common. Check with your dentist if your gums start bleeding or your teeth seem very sensitive.

Animals put down more fat in the skin and abdomen once they've lost their sex hormones; perhaps middle-age spread is the same thing, because about 50% of women around the menopause put on 2.5 kg/5½ lb to 5.0 kg/11 lb in weight.

HOT FLUSHES/NIGHT SWEATS

It seems it's not the actual level of oestrogen in the body, but the sudden fall in levels that give menopausal women hot flushes. The face gets very hot, the neck and face turn red, they start sweating, and the heart beats madly. It can be quite uncomfortable and embarrassing, although it usually only lasts about a minute.

At night you may wake up bathed in sweat and feeling very uncomfortable. It can really disturb your sleep if it happens several times each night. Some women just get the odd flush, some have ten to twenty a day and night. They can start before your periods actually stop, meaning that your ovaries are beginning to wind down.

Until your hormone levels really settle down, your body's temperature control system will be erratic; this can last for months or years. (One in four women get flushes for over five years.) You can help yourself by keeping off tea, coffee and alcohol, all of which may make it worse.

If you're really troubled at night try sleeping in a single bed; you won't be so concerned about disturbing your partner and you will be able to get back to sleep sooner with the bed clothes that are comfortable for you.

If it's really getting you down – feeling embarrassed all the time and tired out from lack of sleep – see what your doctor says about hormone replacement therapy (page 171).

SEX AND REPRODUCTION

As the menopause approaches your period pattern can go haywire – for instance, months without one then a spell of very heavy periods. Make sure you don't get anaemic if this happens to you: feeling very tired even when you wake up in the morning, looking pale, and finding any extra effort difficult, or perhaps making you feel breathless. Your periods become less frequent, with spells of more than a month between them. When a year has gone by without a period the menopause has been reached. Any bleeding after this is taken very seriously (unless it's due to HRT): it can be a sign of early cancer of the uterus (page 61).

Normal oestrogen levels keep the vaginal lining lubricated and resistant to infection. As the oestrogen levels fall after the menopause this can sometimes affect the vagina: it becomes thinner and drier. This can make you feel sore and make you more vulnerable to infections; if you have a discharge or any bleeding tell your doctor. It may make sex uncomfortable; normal lubrication may well be less and you and your partner could end up feeling very sore. Some couples abandon sex altogether at this stage. The problem is easily solved by putting a lubricating jelly (KY) on your partner's penis before intercourse.

Recently, a new product has been released which acts as a vaginal moisturiser (Replens). This cream, which is inserted into the vagina, also makes the vaginal secretions more acid (as in pre-menopause days), which helps combat infection. The cream is effective for seventy-two hours. It's available over the counter at most chemists.

Oestrogen creams strengthen the vaginal lining, but can't be used indefinitely as the hormone is absorbed into the blood stream. If dryness continues to be a problem, HRT can be very helpful.

Some women notice a change in their touch sensation, with feelings of either numbness or oversensitivity. This can happen to the clitoris, making arousal and orgasm difficult or uncomfortable. HRT can also help here if this is a problem.

For many women feelings about sex begin to alter around this time: you may not feel like it so much, you're not turned on as you were before, and your partner may also be having difficulties. There's a lot of things to blame; your hormones, simply being tired and depressed, not talking enough to each other about sex and why it's not right. If your partner feels you don't find him attractive then he won't be able to make love with confidence. Tell him what's going on in your body and in your mind – don't shy away or the problems will grow. If you keep having regular sex, the vagina seems to stay lubricated and stretchy enough. The more you have the better it is.

When can contraception stop?

Although your fertility decreases as the change begins, it only ends with the menopause itself, so it's important to use some form of contraception until then. Pregnancy gets more complicated in your forties with increased miscarriage rate and an increased chance of fetal abnormalities: a mistake at this age could be a disaster.

The problem is knowing when you have had your last period. Safe advice would be to use some form of contraception for two years after the last period for women under fifty, and for one year after the last period in women over fifty. Because of your reduced fertility, the failure rate of various methods of contraception is not so critical. Take advice from your local family planning clinic.

Hormone replacement therapy can't act as a contraceptive but there are new low dose combined pills (Mercilon) that are suitable for fit non-smoking women in their forties.

OSTEOPOROSIS

Our bones are changing from the cradle to the grave. They get bigger until we stop growing, get thicker until we are about forty and then we start to lose bone. Women have less bone than men, and they lose it earlier and faster. Why do women lose bone and where does it go?

Bone is a living substance in which two processes carry on at the same time: one repairing or making new bones, the other removing unwanted bone (the calcium and protein in the bone are absorbed into the blood stream). Our bones get thinner when the removing process takes away more bone than the replacing process: this is called *osteoporosis*, a condition where the bone has become fragile and breaks more easily.

Do thin bones matter?
Yes; the likelihood of breaks and fractures is increased. A seemingly minor fall will result in a broken bone; the hip bone particularly suffers as it is so important in weight bearing. The bones in the spinal column can crack, causing back pain, loss of height and curvature of the spine.

What causes osteoporosis?
Ageing in itself thins the bones of both men and women. But certain things make it worse in women. If our ovaries aren't working properly low oestrogen levels will make us lose bone, whether we are at the menopause or not. If your periods have stopped because of excessive exercise, or undereating (anorexia nervosa, page 21), you may well be thinning your bones. The earlier the menopause starts the greater the risk of osteoporosis. If you've had a hysterectomy while you're still having periods and the ovaries have been removed, your oestrogen levels will be prematurely reduced and put you at risk of osteoporosis. Smokers, because of their earlier menopause, are also at greater risk.

This bone thinning carries on quietly, losing about 2 per cent of your total bone every year after the menopause, without any obvious problems. But it means that the bones are weakened and much more liable to fracture if you fall. More than one in three women will have had a fracture of the wrist or spine by the time they are seventy.

People with severely disabling illnesses, such as rheumatoid arthritis or multiple sclerosis, are more likely to have thin bones, especially if they're being treated with steroids. Anyone who is bedridden for a long time is at a high risk of getting osteoporosis.

How do you know if you've got osteoporosis?
It doesn't show; most people have no idea their bones are thin until they have a fracture, often after the simplest of falls. X-rays show the bones as a greyer colour; normal bone is a bright white.

Tests available

Some hospitals have developed a test (*bone densitometry*) to measure bone mass. It may show if you have thin bones already so that treatment can be started straight away, but it's only a snapshot of your bone at the time and can't predict whether you will lose bone quickly or not. This test is expensive and not widely available.

Blood and urine can be checked for bone hormone levels, and calcium and bone protein levels tests have been developed in Denmark. These may become a much better guide to the rate of bone loss, but they are not in general use in this country at present.

A checklist of risk factors – do these apply to you?

– Being female
– Low oestrogen levels before the menopause: women with irregular or absent periods brought on by excessive exercise, anorexia nervosa, stress
– Women who have had an early menopause (before the age of forty)
– Women who have had their ovaries removed before the menopause
– Thin women: they have less bone to start with and lose it faster
– Family history: if your mother had osteoporosis after the menopause, you're at an increased risk
– White skin: African and Caribbean women seem to have stronger and bigger bones
– Poor diet (calcium deficiency): calcium is needed to build strong bones. When the bone losing process starts in middle age you'll be starting off with strong well-formed bone if your diet has been good: the more you have, the longer it takes to reach fracture risk weakness
– Smokers: these women are usually thinner and have an earlier menopause. Smoking increases bone loss after the menopause
– High alcohol intake: alcohol acts as a bone poison
– Little or no exercise: activity is essential for strengthening your bones, it encourages the bone replacement process. Again, if you build up your bone strength in the first half of your life, the bone loss will take longer to reach osteoporosis levels.

Self-help

The object is to prevent fractures and all the complications they bring. You can make sure your bones are as strong as possible before bone loss begins; you can stop or slow down the bone loss; and you can build up the already thin bones.

DIET Eat a good, well-balanced diet which includes calcium-rich foods (milk, cheese). Many women have low intakes of calcium because they avoid high calorie dairy products. Skimmed and semi-skimmed milk contain the same calcium as full-fat milk and are fine. Calcium supplements are unnecessary if you eat a well-balanced diet and won't prevent bone loss after the menopause. Ideal intake is between 1000 mg and 1500 mg per day for post-menopausal woman. Eating too much protein in your diet increases the loss of calcium; have a well-balanced diet without too much of one type of food (page 11).

Use a fluoride toothpaste, especially if you live in a low fluoride area. Apart from protecting your teeth, fluoride stimulates bone formation (most people ingest small amounts of toothpaste when they're cleaning their teeth). There is concern, however, about using fluoride tablets for any length of time; they may have an adverse effect on bone metabolism after a while.

Calcium supplements have been shown to increase bone density, but only to a modest extent, and certainly not enough to advocate extra calcium for everyone.

CALCIUM CONTENT OF VARIOUS FOODS

Per 100 g	mg calcium	Per 100 g	mg calcium
Milk products		*Bread and grain*	
Butter	15	Bread (white)	50
Cottage cheese	100	Bread (wholewheat)	70
Milk (3.5% fat)	120	Rice (white)	10
Mozzarella cheese	650	Rice (brown)	23
Skimmed milk	130	*Fruit and vegetables*	
Yogurt (low fat)	120	Apple	5
Meat and fish		Orange	40
Beef	8	Prunes	50
Chicken	11	Raisins	80
Cod (fresh)	15	Lettuce	100
Sardines (in oil)	420	Peas	30
Shrimp (cooked)	110	Potatoes	5
Tuna (canned)	8	Tomato	10

EXERCISE It is likely that the major reason for the doubling of the hip fracture rate in the last years has been the fall in physical activity in most women's lives. A fitness plan that involves fairly vigorous exercise three times a week will help to build up your bones (page 12). Moderate exercise of about thirty minutes a day – walking, jogging or dancing – will maintain your bone density when you're past the menopause.

STOP SMOKING Women who smoke are three times more likely to fracture their spines than women who don't smoke. If you are a heavy smoker, stopping smoking can halve the risk of fracture.

HRT and osteoporosis

The most effective way to stop bone loss is hormone replacement therapy (HRT), which contains oestrogen (see opposite). This seems to delay the bone thinning process, which then carries on when the treatment stops.

Research has shown that after stopping HRT bone is lost rapidly, soon reaching levels only slightly better than in women who have never taken HRT. HRT can cut the risk of fracture by half, but it does mean taking long term therapy into your seventies. Many women and their doctors are unhappy about taking prolonged medication for perhaps as long as twenty or thirty years.

What's new

Calcitonin (Calcitare), a hormone produced near the thyroid gland, holds out hope as an alternative to hormone therapy. It also stops the bone removing process. The drug, used for Paget's disease of the bone for many years, is usually administered by injection. A nasal spray has been developed and preliminary work with post-menopausal women is encouraging. It's not available yet on prescription.

Ideally, there should be an easy test to show which women are at risk of losing bone early and fast; for them, HRT, and perhaps calcium supplements, would be highly recommended. Until then, taking regular exercise and, if you smoke, stopping smoking are the most important steps you can take to prevent fractures in old age.

National Osteoporosis Society, PO Box 10, Radstock, Bath BA3 3YB. Tel: 0761 432472.
Women's Health, 52 Featherstone Street, London EC1Y 8RT. Tel: 071–251 6580. Send s.a.e. for publication list.

HORMONE REPLACEMENT THERAPY (HRT)

Hormone replacement therapy became fashionable in America in the sixties and seventies and many women started taking oestrogens in the first rush of enthusiasm. Then it was discovered that a lot of these women were developing cancer of the uterus, many more than would normally be expected. Oestrogen on its own without the natural balance of progesterone could be very dangerous.

Today, HRT has been thoroughly investigated and tested – nobody wants a repeat performance of the cancer scare. Perhaps with this in mind, quite a few family doctors are still unwilling to prescribe it at all. In a recent survey, only 9 per cent of female patients aged between forty and sixty-four were prescribed HRT – more than the previous year, however.

Who needs HRT?

1. Women who for some reason have had their ovaries removed prematurely (a hysterectomy and bilateral hystero-salpingo-oopherectomy).

Oestrogen protects women from heart attacks and strokes, and keeps their bones strong. Take away the hormones and the risk of cardio-vascular disease and osteoporosis increases. Women who have had a hysterectomy, but where the ovaries have been left behind, may also need HRT, as the ovaries sometimes fail earlier than expected.

2. Anyone who is troubled by the symptoms associated with oestrogen deficiency: women who suffer severe hot flushes and night sweats; those with bladder problems; women who have sexual difficulties, such as a dry vagina.

3. Women with arthritis or migraine.

These women may find that things get out of control in the menopause. HRT can stabilise things again.

4. Women who suffer from mood changes, depression and anxiety.

These conditions are difficult to blame on the menopause, but it's worth trying a short course of HRT to see if it's a shortage of hormones that's to blame.

5. Women who have a high risk of heart disease and stroke.

Risk factors include a family history of cardiovascular disease, high blood pressure, a high blood cholesterol count and smoking.

6. Women who have a high risk of getting osteoporosis (page 166).

Who can't have HRT?

1. Women who have had a cancer that's influenced by oestrogens, such as cancer of the breast or uterus.
2. Women who have had trouble with blood clots, particularly those related to pregnancy or the Pill.

HRT can make fibroids bigger and gallstones more troublesome, but these aren't reasons to forbid it, however.

What's available?

HRT normally consists of a mixture of oestrogen and progestogen (a progesterone-like compound). Women who have had a hysterectomy need only take the oestrogen (there's no danger of developing cancer of the uterus).

Oestrogen can be taken by mouth, injected as an implant lasting about six months, or absorbed through the skin from patches.

At the moment progestogen can only be taken by mouth. It's essential to take the progestogen, usually for twelve days each month, to protect the lining of the uterus. It gives you regular lightish periods, although they are not proper periods and they don't mean you're fertile again. Some women suffer mild side-effects, such as breast tenderness, fluid retention and nausea. Most of these symptoms settle down after two or three months. *Any irregular bleeding must be reported straight away.*

HRT is not a contraceptive, the hormone levels are too low. Once you are past the menopause (one year after your last period) HRT doesn't make you fertile again.

TABLETS These come in a calendar pack. The oestrogen is taken every day. The progestogen is taken for twelve days out of the month. Towards the end of the combined tablets you will have a slight bleed.

PATCHES More and more women are taking the oestrogen hormones by applying a skin patch twice a week. Each patch is removed every three to four days and must be put on a hairless area of skin below the waistline. Again, the progestogen tablets need to be taken as above. Soon, it's likely a combined oestrogen and progestogen patch will be available. Some women have a mild skin reaction to the patches.

There are definite advantages in taking oestrogen through a skin patch. In tablet form the oestrogen is absorbed into the intestine and goes straight to the liver. If the hormone goes straight through the skin into the blood stream, the effects on the liver (altering liver enzymes and blood clotting factors) are much reduced.

IMPLANTS A hormone implant consists of a small pellet containing oestrogen which is placed under the skin (usually in the lower abdomen). The skin is numbed with local anaesthetic first, and it takes the doctor about two minutes to put the pellet in place. The pellets usually last six months, but every woman is different. If you've had a hysterectomy this will be all you need; if you haven't, you will need the progestogen tablets as well. When the implant is wearing down you will be aware of a return of your symptoms and you will need to have it replaced.

For how long should it be taken?

If there are good reasons for you starting HRT in the first place and you're quite happy taking it, many experts would say take it indefinitely. At least five years will give your bones a good start in middle age and help to protect your heart and circulation. Remember, HRT is not extra hormones as in the contraceptive Pill – it's replacing your missing hormones and bringing you back to the way you were.

The risks

HRT is not recommended routinely for all women in the menopause. There are always risks attached to any treatment, but given all the information you and your doctor should be able to decide what's best for you.

As breast cancer is encouraged by oestrogens, there are fears that HRT will increase the risk of getting it. Research hasn't confirmed this, but there is evidence to suggest that the risk of breast cancer goes up after treatment for longer than about ten years. Before that, your risk seems to be slightly less than non-takers. However, if you do get breast cancer while taking HRT, your chances of survival are greater than if you were not. To be on the safe side, it's best to examine your breasts regularly and have them checked by your doctor annually. If you have had benign lumps in the breast, or if someone in the family has had breast cancer, it's a good idea to have a mammogram before starting HRT. All women should be invited for a mammogram soon after the age of fifty in any case.

There is no increased risk of cancer of the uterus, ovary or cervix in women who take HRT, in fact it may be lowered.

What's new

A drug called tibolone (Livial) has been recently launched. Its major advantage is that you don't have to have periods at all. You can't start it

173

until you're at least one year beyond your last period. It's good for hot flushes and many of the menopausal symptoms, but it's too early to say whether it will prevent osteoporosis.

> *I had a big operation when I was thirty-nine — I had Crohn's disease, irritable bowel syndrome, which tends to upset everything and accelerate hormone problems.*
>
> *I had terrible problems — huge hormone swings. You feel as though you're going mad. You're very difficult to live with. Enormous tension before a period and my back just knotted up. I had awful problems with back pain.*
>
> *Three years ago I broke my wrist and I began to worry that, like my mother, I had osteoporosis. My doctor sent me to a consultant who said that I did indeed have osteoporosis and at that time I was only forty-six. I saw a female specialist who was wonderful, for the first time I felt my problems were understood.*
>
> *She organised a bone scan and they discovered that my levels were very dangerous. They asked me to consider HRT. I talked it over with my GP and although there were some risks I would rather live with sudden death than my bones wasting away.*
>
> *Three months after I started on HRT my mother died and I was under considerable pressure. Although the HRT was helping it hadn't completely cleared my problems and it was decided I should go on a stronger dose.*
>
> *Now I feel so much better. I think more clearly. I have far greater confidence — and I'm even learning to drive at fifty. I used to really lack self-confidence. My friends tell me I look much better and my back has begun to straighten again.*
>
> *The hot flushes and all those terrible things, they've all gone. I have had no side-effects.*

Women's Health Concern, 83 Earl's Court Road, London W8 6EF. Amarant Trust, 80 Lambeth Road, London SE1 7PW.

URINARY INCONTINENCE

Urinary incontinence can occur at any time but is more common in later life, and understandably many women are too embarrassed even to discuss it with their doctor. This is a shame, because there is plenty on offer in terms of treatment and support. Many hospitals and family doctors have access to a continence adviser trained especially to cope.

There are two main types of incontinence.

Stress incontinence This occurs when pressure brought on by coughing, sneezing or laughing makes urine leak out (it has nothing to do with mental stress).

Urge incontinence This occurs when the bladder loses control and urine is passed regardless of where you are. The bladder is called unstable because it reacts in the wrong way.

It can be difficult to diagnose which type of incontinence is the problem; it is possible to have both. *Urodynamic tests* can help here; these measure how well you pass water, how full your bladder is before you feel the need to go and how well you can control your bladder. This is a painless procedure if a little strange. A catheter (fine tube) is carefully passed into the bladder and then filled with water. The pressure in your bladder throughout the procedure is recorded and the bladder's reaction to the filling is monitored. If you need to go when your bladder has only a small volume in it you may have an urgency problem. After this is finished you are asked to pass urine (in private) into a container which measures the speed of the flow.

Why do women get incontinence?

Incontinence is more common in women; about 10 per cent of young women and 40 per cent of older women have some degree of stress incontinence. In women who have had children, the stretching of muscles and damage to nerves in childbirth can allow the neck of the bladder to drop through the hammock of pelvic floor muscles. When this happens, contracting the pelvic floor isn't effective enough in closing the bladder neck and urine leaks out.

Low levels of oestrogen, around the menopause for example, can upset the bladder making it 'irritable' (urge incontinence) and making the supporting ligaments less strong (stress incontinence).

Some women become bladder obsessed – lying in bed thinking they need to pass urine all the time, always needing to know where the nearest toilet is, and taking every opportunity to go just in case. This encourages an already unstable bladder and makes the condition worse.

Self-help and treatments

PELVIC FLOOR EXERCISES Do these on the hour throughout the day, they will help a great deal to improve strength and reaction time (page 150). Put a finger in the vagina just to make sure you're squeezing the right muscles.

VAGINAL CONES These are a set of equal-sized cones, each a different weight. Starting with a cone weighing 20 g/¾ oz, the woman inserts it into the vagina and keeps it there by tightening the pelvic floor while walking about. She graduates to a heavier cone when she can manage the present one. If this can't be managed it falls out, so it's important to wear underwear. The hospital physiotherapist will give advice on these and help with the exercises.

LOSE WEIGHT Extra weight means extra pressure on the pelvic floor. It probably means you're not taking enough general exercise either. It is difficult to do vigorous exercise if you keep wetting yourself; empty your bladder first and wear a pad. Avoid getting constipated as this can increase the pressure on the bladder.

STOP SMOKING A good hacking smoker's cough is enough to frighten any pelvic floor. It will also undo the good work of any surgery (page 177). Try to stop smoking as soon as you can.

RE-TRAIN THE BLADDER Some women have to go back to something like potty training, and it really helps to have someone like a continence adviser at your local hospital to go to for information and professional support.

Your bladder must be emptied by the clock. Set yourself a target time for a week, say every thirty minutes at first. This means you cannot go to the toilet before the thirty minutes are up; in fact, if you can't wait you must wet yourself. Giving in and going before your target time defeats the object. Surprisingly you won't wet yourself all that often: it's a question of mind over matter.

If you can manage every thirty minutes for a couple of days, increase the target time to every hour and see how you get on. Most people empty their bladders every two or three hours, so once you've reached that you're back to normal.

Re-training your bladder is not as easy as it sounds; some women actually come into hospital for a few days to give it a go: it's called *bladder drill*. There are drugs designed to relax the bladder, such as imipramine (Tofranil) and oxybutynin (Ditropan), and these may be helpful as well. They may cause a dry mouth and blurred vision.

If bed wetting is a problem, try to restrict fluids in the evening. A new spray (Desmospray), containing the artificial hormone desmopressin, reduces urine production for eight to ten hours. It seems to be safe and has no long-term side-effects.

ELECTRICAL THERAPY This is available in some hospitals and works by stimulating the nerves supplying the pelvic floor. A very small electric current is passed through pads attached to the lower abdomen, buttocks or perineum. This makes the woman contract her pelvic floor muscles and strengthens them.

SURGERY If, despite all good intentions and efforts with the pelvic floor, things don't improve, surgery may be considered for stress incontinence to lift up the neck of the bladder. For women with some degree of prolapse (see below), a repair operation is usually done, sometimes with a hysterectomy at the same time. Performed through the vagina, this tightens up the tissues around the bladder neck.

Coping in the meantime

Sanitary pads are not recommended as they are not designed to absorb urine, especially in large quantities. Special pants, designed with a pouch which holds an absorbent pad, are available from an incontinence adviser or larger chemists. These keep the plastic and urine away from the skin, and are very comfortable. High-absorbency pads are also available to wear with normal pants; they can be worn all day without smell or soreness.

Association of Continence Advisers, 380/384 Harrow Road, London W9 2HU. Tel: 071–266 3704.

National Action on Incontinence, 4 St Pancras Way, London NW1 0PE. Send s.a.e to either of these for information on incontinence.

PROLAPSE

This is another problem to do with the pelvic floor, where the uterus or the walls of the vagina come down towards the opening of the vagina. Most women who have a prolapse have had children, so it's assumed that the stretching in childbirth has something to do with it, though occasionally young women who have not had children complain of trouble. Most women with prolapse are over fifty and past the menopause. Losing oestrogen after the menopause makes the ligaments less supple and strong. Being overweight or having a chronic cough all adds extra strain.

DIAGNOSIS Usually a dragging sensation in the pelvis, sometimes worse at period time. You may feel a lump or swelling in the vagina. It's worse when you've been on your feet all day and much better when you've been lying down.

If the front of the vagina is weak, the bladder bulges down (*cystocoele*): this can give you trouble with passing urine and incontinence. If the back wall is weak then the rectum bulges forward, occasionally causing

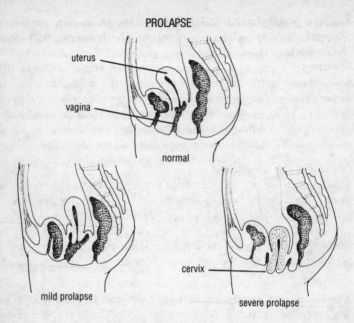

PROLAPSE

uterus

vagina

normal

mild prolapse

cervix

severe prolapse

trouble with the bowel function. You may feel that the vagina is not so tight as it used to be and there may be sexual difficulties if the cervix is low down in the vagina.

TREATMENT It depends whether you can live with it or not. Pelvic floor exercises (page 150) can help but usually if you are having a lot of trouble surgery is the answer. This is a repair operation, sometimes with a vaginal hysterectomy as well. The incision necessary is confined to the vagina so recovery is rapid, much easier than having an abdominal hysterectomy. Sex is fine after everything has healed (usually four to six weeks); it may even be better, because the tissues have been tightened up.

If you're not fit for surgery or it doesn't appeal and you still want some help, a pessary (ring or shelf) can be inserted in the vagina, supporting the uterus. This is changed every three to four months.

Keep doing the pelvic floor exercises!

BREAST PROBLEMS

BREAST CANCER

Many women fear breast cancer most of all the cancers, and it is very common – about one in twelve women will get it. Some women fear the prospect of treatment – often a mastectomy – as much as the cancer itself, but things are changing. Today, early detection and effective treatment mean that women with an early cancer have an 80 per cent chance of being cured.

Who gets breast cancer?

It's much more common in women over the age of fifty and past the menopause, it's rare below thirty. One-third of women are in their seventies when they develop breast cancer, which means the risk for the younger woman is much less (one in 100000 chance in your twenties, rising to one in 1000 risk at the age of forty).

If your mother or sister has had breast cancer then your risk is doubled. It seems that starting your periods early (before twelve) and finishing them late (after fifty) also puts you at a slightly higher risk. Previous surgery for benign breast disease can slightly increase your risk of breast cancer.

Having children, and especially if you have your first child before your thirties, cuts down your risk considerably; this is not enough to advocate all women starting their families early. Japanese women rarely get breast cancer, but if they move to the USA and eat a Western diet, which is high in fat, the chances increase dramatically.

ALCOHOL The evidence is confusing at the moment, with different studies giving conflicting results.

THE PILL AND HRT One study suggested that taking the Pill when relatively young (under twenty-five) or for a long time before a first pregnancy (over four years) may put these women more at risk, but the women in this study were taking higher dose pills than are used these days. Other evidence suggests there's no risk at all, so at the moment there's no clear case against the Pill.

HRT seems to increase your risk of breast cancer if you've been taking it for a long time (about ten years); before that your risk seems to be reduced. If you do develop breast cancer whilst taking HRT your chances of survival are much better compared to women with breast cancer who didn't take HRT.

Where does the cancer come from?

The breast is mainly formed from fatty tissue. It contains milk-producing sacs which drain the milk to the nipple through a system of milk ducts. Cancer can start in the milk sacs or the ducts. The malignant cells behave abnormally and reproduce strangely to form a

BREAST TUMOURS

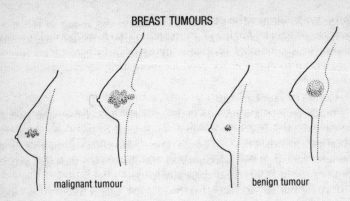

malignant tumour   benign tumour

tumour. The lymphatic system, which runs through the whole body (important in the fight against infection), drains the breast into lymph nodes in the armpit and under the breast bone.

The cancerous cells of a tumour can spread in this lymphatic system to the armpit and chest glands. That's why it's very important to feel in and around your armpits whenever you check your breasts. And that's why surgeons want to know whether the cancer has spread into the glands there.

I can feel a lump – is it cancer?

First, relax. Four out of five lumps are not cancer. If you have been regularly examining your breasts, you will know if it's normal for them to be lumpy occasionally. A suspicious lump is usually painless and can sometimes cause skin puckering or changes in the nipple. Visit your family doctor as soon as possible, you may well be worrying unnecessarily. She will refer you to a hospital breast specialist if there's any doubt. There the lump may be checked to see if it contains fluid, drawing it off with a fine needle and sending it to the laboratory to look for cancer cells. A *mammogram* (X-ray of the breast) may be arranged at the same time.

Taking a small part of the lump (biopsy) is the only way to definitely confirm that it's cancer. This can be done under a local or general anaesthetic. Some surgeons send the tissue for 'frozen' section – this is where the pathologist cuts and freezes the tissue making it easier to examine – which gives an answer in about thirty minutes. If it's positive, the surgeon may remove the breast there and then, although this is less common these days. The more accurate method of examination takes longer, usually a couple of days.

Surgery: what are the options?

Because treatment for breast cancer didn't seem to be making much impact on the number of women dying from breast cancer, surgeons have begun to question the need for mutilating operations like radical mastectomy.

The decision on which treatment is the best for you depends on a variety of factors: your age, whether you are menopausal, the size and position of the tumour, whether there is any spread to the armpit glands or to the chest or bones. Breast cancer is graded in terms of how the disease has spread, from stage one where the tumour is easily movable in the breast, stage two where tumour has spread to the armpit glands, up to stage four where the cancer has spread widely in the body.

MASTECTOMY OPERATIONS

simple mastectomy

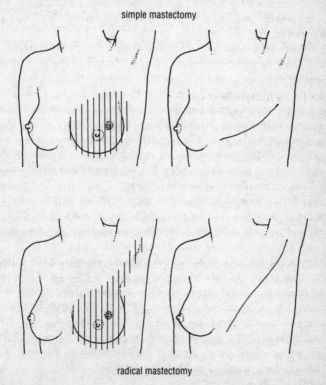

radical mastectomy

LUMPECTOMY

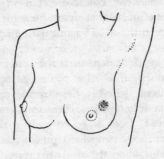

LUMPECTOMY As there's no evidence that mastectomy and more extensive surgery leads to a better survival rate from breast cancer, local removal of tumour has become more popular with surgeons and women alike. However, the less surgery you have the more check-ups you'll need in the future.

Only certain women will be suitable for *lumpectomy* treatment: the tumour must be small, in a readily accessible area of the breast (behind the nipple is difficult) and it mustn't be attached to the muscles under the breast itself. The pathologist must be happy that the tumour is not what is known as an aggressive type. A sample of the armpit glands will be taken as well to see if the disease has spread.

Radiotherapy to the glands in the armpit is necessary as well to reduce the risks of spread. There's a higher risk of the tumour coming back in the same breast – local recurrence – but in terms of survival the outlook is no different from more extensive surgery.

MASTECTOMY A *simple mastectomy* is the removal of the whole breast. A *radical mastectomy* involves the removal of the muscles of the chest wall as well and is rarely done these days (women had a lot of problems after this with arm swelling and limitation of movement).

Mastectomy is the right operation for some women. If the tumour is of a certain type (*multifocal*) or involves a large portion of the breast, mastectomy may be chosen as the best surgical option. Some women may not like the idea of radiotherapy and the small risk of local recurrence with a lumpectomy, and opt for a mastectomy.

A recent study has suggested that if you have breast cancer while still having periods, you have a much better chance of survival if your operation is done in the second half of the cycle.

Are there any further treatments?

Further treatment may be considered when the pathologist has examined the tumour and the sample of armpit glands. Tamoxifen (Nolvadex) is a drug that works against your natural oestrogens. It's used in the treatment of advanced breast cancer and improves survival. It may also be used in addition to surgery in premenopausal women in whom the disease has spread.

Chemotherapy (for example, cyclophosphamide) may also be necessary; it has side-effects like loss of hair and nausea, but these improve once the treatment stops.

Whatever happens you will need to be followed up closely afterwards and you will need to be seen more regularly the less surgery you have.

Making a decision about treatment

Women who are offered a choice between mastectomy and lumpectomy are less anxious and depressed than those offered no choice. If this problem is facing you, don't be hurried into a decision because you've got cancer and feel something must be done immediately.

Talk it over with your consultant surgeon; ask him (it's nearly always a man) if he has a specialist breast nurse attached to his team whom you can see. She will have more time to outline in detail what the treatment will involve. If you're really unhappy about the options on offer ask your family doctor to arrange a second opinion, most consultants don't mind about this.

It's very important to know what's going on, be involved in the decision-making and accept the treatment that's chosen. Being in control is vital to your recovery and future quality of life.

BREAST RECONSTRUCTION

Depending on the particular case some women are suitable for the creation of a new breast. This has to be discussed fully with your surgeon; sometimes it's possible to have a *subcutaneous mastectomy* which removes the entire breast tissue but leaves the skin and nipple intact, and then a silicone implant is put in the cavity.

Breast reconstruction sometime after a mastectomy involves transferring tissue from other areas of the body (back muscle, abdominal muscle, skin and fat) and is more complicated. Nipple formation is done usually as a separate operation using ear or inner thigh tissue and sometimes some nipple skin from the other breast. There are complications with all plastic surgery (ranging from infection, bleeding and scarring to rejection of the implant) which you must be aware of before you embark on more surgery.

Surgeons don't think there is a danger of missing any returning tumour under the implant; regular examination and mammography should pick it up early.

Some women mourn the loss of a breast and, despite the surgery, with it's complications and often imperfect results (ask your surgeon if you can see some before and after photographs), are desperate to feel normal again, going to any lengths to achieve this. Your partner may play a big part in this; talk about this in detail together if you're considering breast reconstruction.

Prosthesis

After a mastectomy operation you will leave hospital with a temporary lightweight breast form (*prosthesis*) to wear for the first few weeks. A month or two later a permanent prosthesis will be fitted which is made of moulded silicone.

BREAST CANCER AND THE MIND

There is a great deal of psychological trauma associated with the diagnosis of breast cancer. We live in a world of the bosom, where the female form is forced upon us everywhere to sell everything. The loss of a breast or conservative treatment for breast cancer can affect the way a woman thinks about herself and her sexuality, and if she's dissatisfied with herself, her self-esteem goes down.

Some women think they're not sexually attractive anymore – they may reject their partners for fear of being rejected first. Communications may break down. Studies have shown that a good proportion of women following mastectomy were still having psychological and sexual problems one to two years later.

Husbands and partners, too, can have a tough time. Men often feel helpless and don't know how best to support their partners. They need reassurance and guidance as well. Help is available from the specialist breast nurse or your family doctor.

Recent research has found that stress can contribute to the recurrence of breast cancer. Those women who had experienced a 'severe life event' (divorce, family death) were almost six times more likely to have a recurrence. A small American study found better survival rates in women who had psychotherapy after treatment than those who had no support. The psychotherapy involved airing of feelings, establishing emotional bonds with fellow sufferers and learning to cope with cancer. Whether or not this work will be confirmed on a larger scale has yet to be seen, but the idea of some organised psychotherapy or counselling for women recovering from breast cancer makes good sense.

Can I prevent it happening to me?

Some interesting animal studies have shown that a high fibre, low fat diet seems to protect against breast cancer. Alcohol is shown to increase your risk in some studies but not in others. Tamoxifen, the drug used for breast cancer, has been given to healthy women in a ten-year study to see if it could actually prevent it; the study is only half finished but the results look promising.

Another drug (gestodene) which is the progestogen part of some newer oral contraceptives also looks as though it could prevent the disease developing (it's a possibility that the newer Pills could actually help to prevent breast cancer).

Finding the cancer early gives you the best chance of a cure. Examining your breasts every month (page 34) is vital as is taking up the offers of mammography for women over fifty (page 36).

I found a lump through self examination on my breast – I usually test after a period. (I still have my period.) I felt worried straight away because my mother died of tummy cancer. I phoned the doctor straight away, and got an appointment the next day. He examined me and said it didn't seem too bad but referred me to the specialist.

I went to see a gynaecologist because I had an anaemia problem, and I asked him to look at it because I was so worried. He looked at it, and asked if I would like him to hurry the process up. He arranged for me to see a specialist the next day at the hospital.

The specialist knew straight away to remove the lump and made an appointment for me to have it removed the following week. It was removed while I was under general anaesthetic, and I stayed overnight. It took ten days before the stitches were ready to be removed, and when I went in they had the results back. I was told it was a growth, and that they had removed a lot of the surrounding tissue. They said I would have to have radiotherapy.

Six weeks later when the wound had healed, I had radiotherapy five days a week for five weeks, at five minutes a time. I didn't suffer from any side-effects so I carried on working. The nurses did the radiotherapy – they were excellent people, kind and thoughtful. The consultant came in every so often.

I went once a month for six months to see the consultant and to be examined, then every two months for six months, and finally every three months. And now I will go every four months. They will keep seeing me for ten years, at regular intervals, and if I'm worried they will see me.

Breast Care and Mastectomy Association (BCMA), 26 Harrison Street, Kings Cross, London WC1H 8JG. Tel: 071–867 1103. Offers information and support to women with breast cancer and their friends and families.

Women's National Cancer Control Campaign, Suna House, 128–130 Curtain Road, London EC2A 3AR. Tel: 071–729 2229 (see page 36). Information and advice on screening and early detection of breast cancer.

Breast Care Campaign Helpline. Tel: 0628 481233, 5pm–8pm. Helpline for women worried in general about their breasts.

BENIGN BREAST DISEASE

For some women lumpy breasts are the norm. The condition is sometimes called *fibrocystic disease* (or benign breast disease) and involves extra growth in certain parts of the breast: the fibrous supporting tissue and the glandular milk-producing cells.

This can mean the lumpy texture of the breasts, which many women feel before their periods, doesn't go away. It's thought the breasts are for some reason particularly sensitive to oestrogen and progesterone, which encourages growth of certain breast tissues.

BREAST CYSTS

These are usually caused by a block in the drainage of fluid due to the stimulation of the glandular milk-producing cells. A breast specialist will suggest draining by piercing through the skin with a fine needle and drawing off the fluid, which is then sent off to check for cancer cells as a precaution. If the lump disappears then all's well, if it doesn't further tests may be necessary.

BREAST LUMPS

A collection of fibrous tissue can sometimes cause a lump (*fibroadenoma*, called a breast mouse because it appears to move freely when examined).

You will need to be seen by a breast specialist who may recommend a mammogram, take a small portion of the tissue for analysis (biopsy) or remove the whole lump.

BREAST PAIN

This is rarely breast cancer. Nevertheless, it can be very distressing and uncomfortable. It's sometimes cyclical, worse before a period, or bear no relation to anything.

Treatment is similar to that for PMS with evening primrose oil (Efamast, treatment needs to be continued for at least two months before any benefit) and hormone therapy (danazol – Danol, dydrogesterone – Duphaston or the Pill). Bromocriptine, a drug that lowers *prolactin* (a hormone produced by the pituitary gland and which controls breast activity), can work very well for some women.

INDEX

Other titles available from BBC Books: